Paula Horan

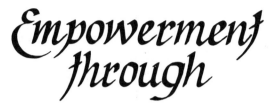

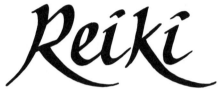

The path to personal
and global transformation

LOTUS LIGHT
SHANGRI-LA

Special Notice

Although this book offers a variety of tools for healing and self-transformation, it is not meant to give recommendations or advice for the treatment of specific illnesses. It is suggested that you consult a physician or qualified wholistic health practitioner before pursuing any form of therapy.

Paula Horan, Ph.D.

1st English edition 1990
2nd English edition 1993
3rd English edition 1993
4th English edition 1994
5th English edition 1994
6th English edition 1995
7th English edition 1996
8th English edition 1997
9th English edition 1998
10th English edition 2000
11th English edition 2002

Lotus Press
P.O. Box 325, Twin Lakes, WI 53181

The Shangri-La series is published
in cooperation with Schneelöwe Verlagsberatung,
Federal Republic of Germany
Originally published 1989,
© by Schneelöwe Verlagsberatung,
87648 Aitrang, Federal Republic of Germany
All rights reserved
Cover design and illustration: Wolfgang Jünemann
Illustrations by Peter Ehrhardt

ISBN 0-941524-84-1
Printed in the USA

*This book is dedicated
to all those in search
of greater emanence*

e · mi · nence ('em – – – nen (t) s) . n 1: a position of prominence or superiority – used as a title for a cardinal. 2: something eminent, prominent, or lofty: as a: a person of high rank or attainments b: a natural elevation. Webster's

em · a · nate ('em – – – nat) vb – nat ed: nat-ing {L. emanatus, pp. of emanare, fr. e – t manave to flow] vi: to come out from a source vt: to give out : EMIT syn. Webster's

es · sence (es' ns) , 1: that by which a thing is what it is; intrinsic nature; important that is, csp, a spiritual or immaterial entity. The American College Dictionary

The above three are the triune aspect of Emanence – a word coined by the author to illustrate the coming together of the presently triune aspect of man. Similarly in hermetic science, the first three laws represent the triune aspect of what is really one absolute law. Man has experienced this law through what might be described as a triangular "prism" due to the veils over consciousness which block a clear perception of truth. At the current point in history in which humanity is undergoing a baptism by fire – the fire of love which purifies mind, we are seeing the resulting effect of these veils being lifted away and the state of Emanence made manifest.

e · ma · nence ('em – – – nen (t) s n. the state of a person who through his inner work to develop consciousness, has reached a deeper level of communication, and thus a higher standing with his Higher (Universal or God) self. The resulting level of conscious awareness in turn produces a higher vibratory frequency which issues forth to those around him. This is felt by others as the emanation of Love energy – the core of substance of oneself. Author

4

Table of Contents

Foreword

This book shares the deepest public understanding of Reiki that I have ever seen. I believe this is because Paula Horan, a Ph.D. psychologist, is approaching it from the reference point of an accomplished and holistic healer, as a person deeply involved in her own spiritual development, as well as a Reiki Master. It is also this background and consciousness that allows her to rise above the dualism of the different Reiki schools to celebrate the eternal principles of Reiki.

As she elucidates the way that Reiki works to heal on the physical, subtle, and causal levels one begins to see the important link that she makes between Reiki and all other forms of healing and spiritual unfoldment. From my work as a wholistic physician, Reiki master, director of the Tree of Life Seminars, co-director of the first Kundalini Clinic in the United States, and author of *Spiritual Nutrition and the Rainbow Diet*, I want to completely validate her findings. Her understanding is synchronous with that put forth in my book which is that we are composed of more solid energy fields, which we call the physical body and less dense fields, which I call subtle organizing energy fields(SOEFs). These SOEFs are moving faster than the speed of light and also simultaneously slower than the speed of light, reflecting the multidimensionality of the human condition. These SOEFs act as vortexes for the faster than the speed of light cosmic energy to come into the body, which is slower than the speed of light dimension, and also act as templates for the structure and function of the emotional, mental, and physical body. On the physical level, when these SOEFs are filled with energy they become well organized. As part of a step down template phenomena, they create a well organized DNA/RNA system, which in turn creates well functioning enzymes, protein synthesis, and cell division. When the cells divide and function well, then the glands, organs, and tissues function well and we have health.

Conversely, when the SOEFs lose energy, and become disrupted through the stress of emotional mental, spiritual, or poor life style imbalances, they act as poor templates for the physical functioning and we get disease. The process of SOEF loss of energy and disorganization is the process of aging, or in terms of Second Law of Thermodynamics, it is an increase in entropy. The process of increasing the energy and therefore the organization of the SOEFs is the process of growing younger; it is a process of healing. According to the Second Law of Thermodynamics, it is reversing entropy. Reiki directly brings in the universal life force to the SOEFs, which directly energizes them and consequently organizes them. In other words, Reiki reverses the aging process by reversing the increase in entropy. It does this directly, and also indirectly by rebalancing the subtle bodies and chakras. When the subtle bodies and chakras are not aligned, they block the incoming universal life force into the human system. Once aligned, the energy flows freely. This results in a reversal of entropy and therefore healing on an emotional, mental, and spiritual level. Once the reader understands this simple concept, it is easier to appreciate the depth of Paula's book.

Paula's point that to learn Reiki does not require months of study, or even an intellecutal understanding, although some of us always enjoy doing that, is very important. The beauty of Reiki lies in its simplicity. Reiki is the democratization of the healing process. This book and Ms. Horan's teaching Reiki in Third World countries is part of that process. Reiki is Divine grace meant for anyone who is open to receiving it.

This book deepens the understanding of another point that is significant. It is that Reiki aids everyone along the spiritual continuum. Again, my observations with students directly support Paula's findings. After the Reiki initiations there seems to be an accelerated spiritual jump. I regularly see a variety of emotional and spiritual breakthroughs after initiations. Often there is also a great deal of spontaneous joy that people begin to experience after an initiation, and which continues if they keep up the practice of the self-healing aspect of Reiki. I appreciate her focus on the 21 day healing cycle because it helps us take note of it as a specific time period so students can better be aware of it.

If one understands, as I have scientifically demonstrated in *Spiritual Nutrition and the Rainbow Diet*, that we humans are human crystals made of a series of oscillating solid and liquid crystals, then Paula's findings have a conceptual explanation on a vibratory level. Dissonant thoughts and negative thoughts or emotions have a lower vibration in our crystalline structure; with Reiki the vibration rate is raised toward our full potential. It becomes so strong that the crystallized denser thoughtforms are not able to sustain their local locus of dissonance and become broken up and released from our physical or subtle bodies. If we are able to just observe them and release them rather than get involved with them, they leave our total system. I have also observed this same process happens for meditators as well. Once these points of dissonance are forced out of the system, the overal crystalline structure of our system becomes more resonant and the universal life force moves more freely. The more the life force energy is free to move in the body, the easier it is for the kundalini, the spiritually transformative energy, to be awakened. Once the kundalini is awakened, this release of emotional and mental blocks is even more accelerated. Reiki is not only a democratization of the ability to heal and self-heal, but it also makes a level of spiritual transformation available to non-meditators, that is usually reserved for those with a meditative path.

Throughout this book, Paula writes with such a joyful creativeness and love for Reiki, that it is easy to follow her in the application of Reiki into many forms of healing and life situations. One may wonder, for example, how a Reiki treatment can speed up the detoxification during a fast or if it really works on mechanical devices that have broken down. It does. For example, on a European workshop tour, may wife got stuck in a bathroom in a museum in Geneva, Switzerland. The lock had jammed. One of our group went to get the caretaker. I applied Reiki to the lock while we were waiting. After a few minutes the lock unjammed and she was rescued from the clutches of the bathroom. In my spiritual fasting retreats we use a form of group Reiki and crystal healing that seems to accelerate the detox process and minimize the detox reactions of fasting. The reason for this is that the ability to detox, as the toxemia expert, Dr. Tilden has pointed out, is dependent on the vitality of the body. If there is greater vitality or life force, then the body can better function to detox itself. Reiki treatments increase the vitality and therefore enhance the ability of the body to detox.

This book gives a wonderful and penetrating insight into the inner process of Reiki that is useful for experienced Reiki teachers as well as for the lay public. Because of Paula's extensive experience as a healer and indepth understanding of healing, she is able to point toward some unitive understandings which give some insight into the workings of Reiki and of some general principles of healing itself. As Reiki is a form of grace for all who use it, this book comes through as a form of grace for all who read it.

Gabriel Cousens, M.D., Reiki Master

Acknowledgements

This book is part of an ongoing process which I began 23 years ago in the pursuit of viable self-healing methods. My early adventures in curing grand mal epilepsy, fibrous cysts, and tumors, helped to teach me of the power of mind when integrated with matter and of other subtle bodies beyond the realm of the visible. Although our higher self is our own best teacher, there are always those along the path who help to guide and enrich us with their knowledge and experience.

I have been blessed with many excellent teachers too numerous to mention, however I would like to thank the faculty and staff of The University for Humanistic Studies and the Institute of Psycho-Structural Balancing in San Diego for their love and support.

Special recognition is due to the following people whose specific ideas are included in this book: Paavo Airola, Vicki and Randall Baer, Ken Dychtwald, Eugene Ferson, Bara Fischer, Leonard Orr, Joyce Nelson, John Randolph Price, Sondra Ray, Ida Rolf, William Tiller, and Marcel Vogel.

I would also like to thank my own Reiki Master Kate Nani of San Diego, and those who have trained in Third Degree with me for their help in spreading the Reiki energies around the world: Don Riches of London, Glen of Trees of New York, Nari Mayo of Phoenix, Trina McAtee of Colorado Springs, Francine Timothy of Paris, France, Karl Everding of Frankfurt, Brigitte Ziegler of Munich, Barbara Szepan of Siegsdorf, Helga Zepeck-Zimmermann of Munich, Regina Wagner of Hannover, Germany, Gudrun Óladóttir of Reykjavik, Iceland, Judit Erdész, Erzséberszabo, and Andrea Golzo of Budapest, Hungary and Dwayne JaQuenex of Portland, Oregon.

I give special thanks to Nari Mayo for permission to use her poems and figure drawings; to my father Robert Horan for his support in furnishing me with a quiet place to write and a base for my European efforts; and very special thanks to Dwayne JaQue-nex for his work on the Macintosh, his expert graphic layout and extensive editing, without which this book would not have had such a wonderful flow.

Finally, I would like to acknowledge all of my students for their encouragement on this project, and to you the reader for persisting in your goal toward personal transformation.

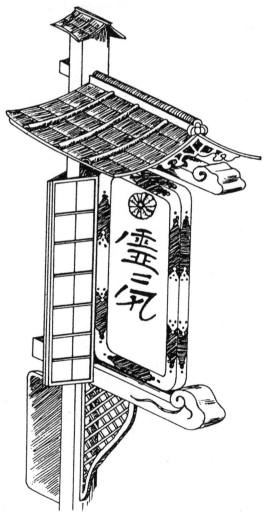

INTRODUCTION

Currently, there is a great need shown in societies around the world, for a healing of the inner self, the need to become unified or whole, in short to reach a state of Emanence.

Two thousand years ago man began to be initiated by water as is seen by the voice crying out in the wilderness, John, who baptized humanity with water. The purpose of the water initiation was to cleanse and regenerate our bodies – our physical and animal natures – so that we could then properly receive "higher vibratory" teachings. This initiation had a powerful effect on mankind. Our philosophy changed from one of "eye for an eye, tooth for a tooth," as seen in the Old Testament, to one of "turning the other cheek" as promoted in the New Testament and demonstrated by Ghandi and Martin Luther King in recent times.

Old habits die hard, and although many positive changes have occurred, wars at present cover large areas of the planet, the distribution of goods is completely out of balance, and the overwhelming disregard for ecology through the current destruction of the planet is the present state of affairs. It is quite apparent that politics and religion cannot provide all of the answers. Only a total quantum leap in the consciousness of mankind will provide the cure. Although the water initiation moved us ahead quite quickly and opened us up to new possibilities, we are still in need of a profound mental purification.

Now, twenty centuries later, we are receiving the fire initiation. Humanity is currently receiving a baptism by fire, the purification of the human mind through knowledge aflame with Love. This knowledge may come through conscious effort, or when laws are transgressed, nature may teach us through forest fires, chemical fires, nuclear accidents, etc. Note the number of fiery disasters which have occurred in the past couple of years.

This initiation by fire is the preparation for the next initiation by Spirit. According to Hermetic Science, man will not realize

Spirit until his body is made clean by water, and his mind pure by fire. In other words, no man will be liberated from the bonds of fear and ignorance, and raise his level of conscious awareness, who has not regenerated his body through Life Energy, and purified his mind by Truth and Love.

There are many paths to purification resulting in a state of Emanence, indeed there are as many paths as there are people on the planet. Disease in my own body, specifically a past history of grand mal epilepsy, and breast tumors, in retrospect, has been a fortunate path, as it has helped me to engage in a journey toward wholeness, which involved me in the study of several healing modalities. As a result I discovered the power of the mind integrated with matter and the extreme importance of diet. My studies also led me to explore and master several of the mind/body therapies, which ultimately led me further into research of the more phenomenal psychic healings in Mexico and Brazil.

Then I encountered Reiki. Nowhere have I found a simpler, more profound method to help someone heal the Body/Mind/Spirit to a state of wholeness and balance, resulting in the experience of Emanence.

This book is primarily a book about Reiki, designed to appeal to both the uninitiated layman and the experienced Reiki practitioner. There is however a wealth of information laced between the Reiki material, which I have gleaned from my years of research in the healing field. In addition, due to my background as a psychologist, I have included information on body psychology to help practitioners understand some of the causal levels of dis-ease, which are linked to the specific areas in which energy blocks are found. I have also included a list of books I recommend to further aid in your exploration of the healing field.

This book is dedicated to my Reiki students all over the world who have graced me with the privilege of helping them "fine tune" to greater degrees of Emanence. I offer you my sincere gratitude for having given me the additional privilege of directly experiencing your Higher Selves during the attunement process.

14

You have all helped me to reconfirm the truth of our union in one Universal Spirit. This book will hopefully help to reconfirm that truth in you. I've written this book also to inspire you to continue in your work toward greater conscious awareness, perhaps reminding you along the way of things you might have temporarily forgotten. I wish you Love, Light, and further Emanence.

Paula Horan

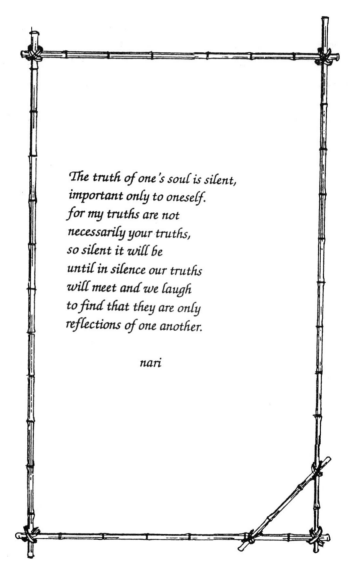

The truth of one's soul is silent,
important only to oneself.
for my truths are not
necessarily your truths,
so silent it will be
until in silence our truths
will meet and we laugh
to find that they are only
reflections of one another.

nari

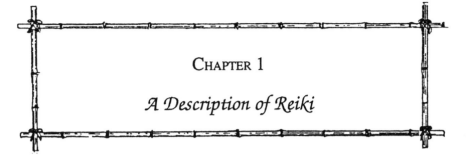

CHAPTER 1

A Description of Reiki

Reiki is the Japanese word for Universal Life Force Energy. When the 'Rei' and 'Ki' are broken down into their two component parts, the Kanji (Japanese alphabet) definition for Rei is universal, transcendental spirit, mysterious power, essence. Ki is described as the vital life force energy, very similar to the Chi of Chinese acupuncture, Light to Christians, and Bioplasmic Energy to Russian researchers.

We all have Reiki energy (Universal Life Force Energy), for it is our birthright. What makes Reiki different from other healing methods, is the attunement (also known as the initiation) process which the student experiences in the various levels of Reiki classes. Anyone can lay their hands on another person and help accelerate the healing process by transferring magnetic energy. A person who has been through the process of Reiki attunements however, has experienced a very ancient technology for fine tuning the physical and etheric bodies to a higher vibratory level. In addition, certain of the energy centers, also known as chakras, are opened to enable the person to channel (and vibrate) higher amounts of Universal Life Force Energy.

Reiki is never sent, it is drawn through the channel. For example, if I lay my hands on you to do a treatment, you will draw appropriate amounts of energy to which ever areas of your body need it. I am never drained in the process, as I too am treated as I "give" a treatment. The energy enters at my crown chakra and passes through the upper energy centers to my heart and solar plexus. The rest then passes through my arms and hands to your body. I am thus never drained in the process, as a certain amount of energy is stored in me. However, at the same time, you do not take on any of my "stuff" (negative energy or blocks) as the Reiki passes through a purified channel in my body, opened by the attunements.

One of the greatest benefits of Reiki is the possibility of self-treatment. Once a person is attuned, he or she need only have the intention to do Reiki on him/herself or others and the energy is immediately drawn through.

Self-treatment is an extremely effective technique for total relaxation and stress release. It amplifies the life force energy in our body which then helps create balance in the physical and etheric bodies. Treating oneself also helps to release withheld emotions and energy blocks.

Reiki is not a religion, as it holds no creed or doctrine. Indeed, it is a very ancient science hidden for thousands of years, until Dr. Usui rediscovered this very old "technology" hidden in the Tibetan Sutras. Researchers at Stanford, using highly sensitive instruments, which measure the flow of energy forces entering the body, determined that Reiki energy enters the healer through the top of the head (or crown chakra) and exits through the hands. The energy force comes from a northerly direction, but from the south when below the equator. In addition, once the Reiki energy is activated, it seems to flow in a counterclockwise spiral motion, much like the double helix in DNA.

The amount of energy emanating from the hands definitely increases during treatment. Dr. Bara Fischer, of Santa Fe, New Mexico, a well-known researcher who has developed an ingenious technique for doing life-energy interpretations with Kirlian photography, tested the author before and during the sending of an absentee healing. The photograph taken during the absentee healing displayed a marked increase of radiation when compared with the photo taken before the treatment, which had displayed a definitively smaller range of emanations.

The evidence to date shows very clearly that there is indeed a plasmatic streaming – a release of energy through the bodily

18

system – when blocks are released. All outcomes are different for every treatment, the healee being the determining factor in the net result. Each person draws in just the right amount of life force that he or she needs to release, activate, or transform the energy of the physical and etheric bodies. Reiki not only can effect change in the chemical structure of the body, by helping to regenerate organs and rebuild tissue and bone, it also helps create balance on the mental level. Reiki is not a belief system, therefore no mental preparation or direction is needed to receive a treatment, only a desire to receive and accept the energy. On the other hand, from the standpoint of the practitioner, since it is not a belief system, once the intention is clear to start a treatment, it will always be activated when used as instructed.

Reiki is a wonderful tool to help one develop conscious awareness, the very key to enlightenment. As in most things in life, Reiki must be experienced to be appreciated. May your exploration of Reiki be a joyous one!

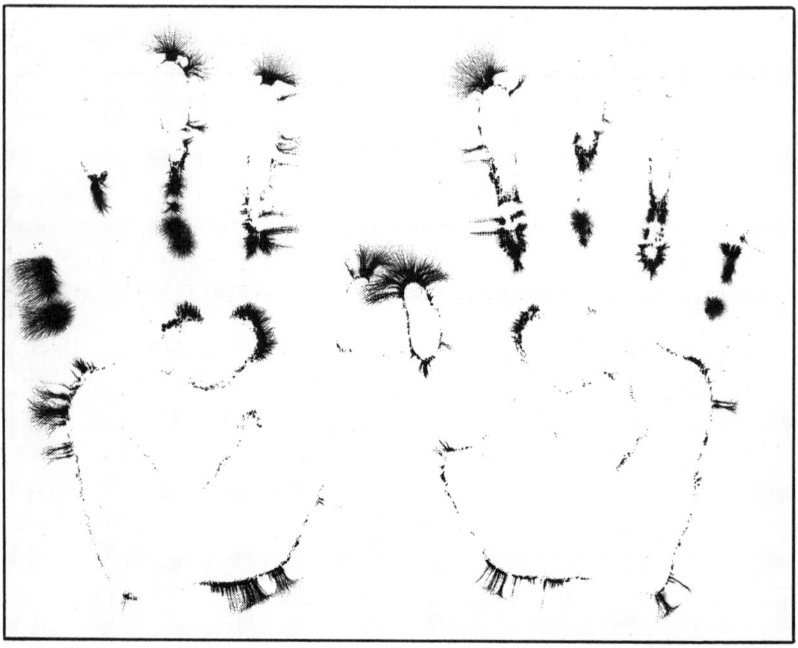

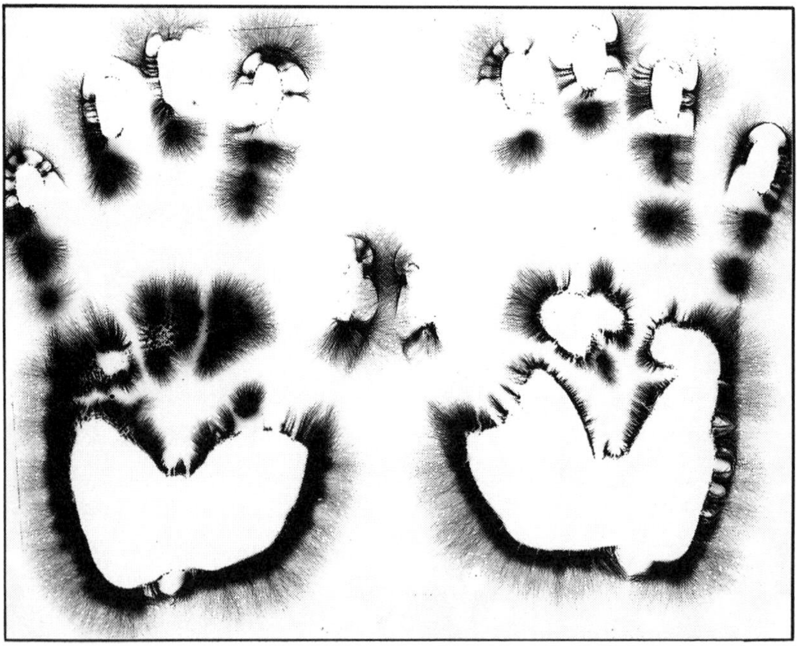

CHAPTER 2

The History of Reiki

During the middle of the Meiji era in Japan, which covers the mid-1800's, Dr. Mikao Usui was the Dean of a small Christian University in Kyoto. This was an exciting period in Japan's history and many changes were occurring throughout society. The Japanese had only recently reopened their shores to the "barbarian" foreigners, and were quickly adopting all of the new technology of the industrial revolution. Railroads were being built, and even American baseball entered the scene. Along with the return of our diplomats, the Christian missionaries had also returned and spawned a new interest in the already eclectic Japanese (many Japanese celebrate Shinto weddings and are buried in Buddhist ceremonies). Dr. Usui however, had adopted Christianity wholeheartedly, becoming a minister and then finally Dean of a Christian seminary.

One day, during a discussion with some of his students, Usui was asked if he believed literally in the Bible. When he replied that he did, his students reminded him of the instant healings of Christ. The students mentioned that in the Bible, Christ states, "You will do as I have done, and even greater things. If this is so," they stated, "Why aren't there many healers in the world today performing the same acts as Christ? In addition, he tells the apostles to heal the sick and raise the dead. If this is true," the students said, "please teach us the methods." Usui was stunned. In traditional Japanese style, he was bound by his honor as Dean, to be able to answer their questions. On that day Usui resigned his position, and determined to find the answers to this great mystery. As most of his teachers had been American missionaries,

21

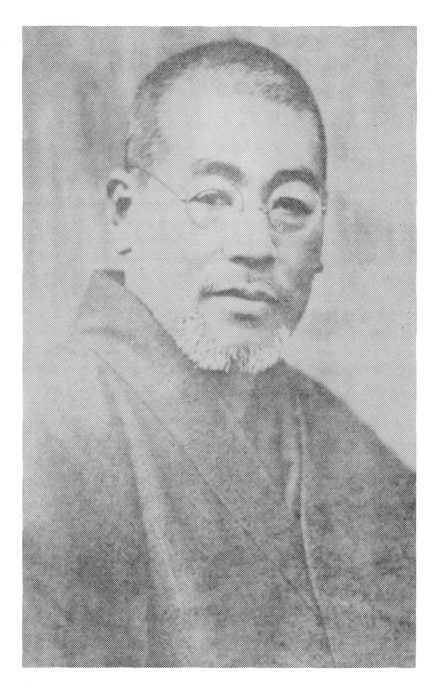

and America was predominantly a Christian country, he decided to begin his study at the University of Chicago in the theological seminary. After a long period of study, in which he did not find his answers, Usui resolved to continue his research elsewhere. Dr. Usui realized that Buddha was also known to have performed incredible healings, so he determined to return to Japan, and see if he could indeed find some "new" old information about more of the instantaneous types of physical healings. Even if all records of the how and wherefores of Christ's healings had been lost, perhaps he might find information about Buddha's healings in the Japanese Lotus Sutras. Upon his return, Usui began an investigation of several Buddhist monasteries. Each time he approached the abbots of the various monasteries asking: "Do you have any records of Buddha's healings of the body?", he received a similar reply, that all focus was now placed on the healing of the Spirit. Usui was determined in his search, and after many tries he came upon a Zen monastery, where for the first time he was encouraged to continue in his search. The old abbot agreed that it must be possible to heal the body, as Buddha had indeed done, but that for centuries all concentration had been focused on healing the Spirit. He stated that "Whatever was possible at one time, can be accomplished again. Perhaps you should stay here and continue your quest," said the abbot. Usui was greatly inspired by the abbot's enthusiasm and began a long study of the Sutras in Japanese. When the results were not forthcoming, he began an indepth study of Chinese, and later covered as much of the Chinese Sutras as he could find. Once again, with little new information being revealed, Usui determined to study the Sutras of Tibet. To do this he required a knowledge of Sanskrit, the next study, which he gladly pursued. It is very likely that shortly after this time he made his trip to northern India, to the Himalayas. During the last century, Tibetan scrolls were found that document the travels of St. Isa, which several scholars feel was actually Jesus. Whether Usui found these same scrolls, or perhaps some other ancient scrolls with the recordings of certain healings, is not known. What we do know is that after completing his study of the Tibetan Lotus Sutras, Usui felt that he had found the intellectual answers to the healings of Christ. What he needed then was the empowerment.

Realizing that he had found the key to the healings, Usui went back to his friend the abbot to ask for advice on how to receive the actual empowerment. They both began to meditate, and together came to the conclusion that Dr. Usui should proceed to a sacred mountain about 17 miles from Kyoto, Mount Kuri Yama, and commence a 21 day fast and meditation, very much like an American Indian vision quest.

Soon after, Usui began his pilgrimage up the mountain. He came to a specific spot facing east, and gathered up a pile of 21 stones which would be his calendar. After 20 days of fasting he arrived at the predawn of the 21st day. As it was the time of the new moon, it was quite dark when he felt around for his last stone. Nothing out of the ordinary had occurred up to this point. He prayed for the answer to come. Out of the sky he saw a flicker of light appear. It began to move very rapidly toward him. As it came closer it also got larger. Usui began to get frightened. He felt like getting up and running away. Finally he realized this must be some sort of sign. He had sought so long and hard all of those years – he just couldn't give up. He girded himself for whatever might come, and momentarily the light struck him in the center of his forehead. Usui thought he had died. Millions of rainbow colored bubbles appeared before his eyes. Soon they became white glowing bubbles, each one containing a three-dimensional Sanskrit character in gold. They would appear one by one, just slowly enough for him to register each character. Finally, when it felt complete, Usui was filled with gratitude. As he had been in a trance-like state, he was surprised when he awakened and it was broad daylight. In his excitement to share his experience with his old friend the abbot, Usui began to run down the mountain. He was amazed at how strong and rejuvenated he felt, considering the long fast he had just completed. This was the first "miracle" of the morning. Suddenly, in his haste, he tripped and stubbed his toe. As he instinctively reached down to grab it, he was amazed that in a few short minutes, the bleeding had stopped and it had completely healed – the second miracle of the morning. As he continued down the mountain, he came to a typical roadside stand, and proceeded to order a full breakfast. As anyone knows, who is acquainted with fasting procedures, it is quite dangerous to break a long fast with a large meal. The proprietor could see by Usui's monk's garb, and unkempt beard, that he had been fasting and meditating, and encouraged him to instead have some special broth. Usui declined and ordered the full breakfast. The third "miracle" of the morning occurred when he ate it without indigestion.

As it turned out, the old man's granddaughter who served Usui, was in dire pain. She had a severe toothache and her jaw had been swollen for days. Her grandfather was too poor to take her to a dentist in Kyoto, so when Usui offered to try and help, she gladly accepted. After he put his hands on the sides of her face, the fourth "miracle" occurred, as the pain and swelling began to disappear.

Dr. Usui then continued on his way back to the monastery. He found the abbot in great pain with a bout of arthritis. While Usui shared his experiences with the monk he laid his hands on the arthritic areas, and very quickly, the pain disappeared. The old abbot was truly amazed. Usui sought his advice as to what he should do with this new found ability. He was again encouraged to meditate, and finally after some discussion, he decided to go and work in the Beggars Quarter of Kyoto. He hoped to heal the beggars so that they could receive new names at the temple, and thus be reintegrated into society.

When Usui entered the Beggars Quarter, he set about immediately, healing young and old alike. The results were remarkable and many received complete healings. After about seven years of this work, Usui began to notice familiar faces. One young man, who looked especially familiar, drew his attention. "Don't I know you?" he asked.

"Why certainly!" he replied, "I'm one of the first people you healed, I received a name, I found a job, and even married. I just couldn't stand the responsibility. It's much easier to be a beggar."

Usui soon found many similar cases. In despair he wept. Where had he gone so wrong? It finally dawned on him that he had failed to teach them responsibility, and most of all, gratitude. He then realized that the healing of the Spirit was every bit as important as the healing of the body. He saw that by having given Reiki away he had further impressed the beggar pattern in them. The importance of an exchange of energy became clear to him. People needed to give back for what they received or life would be devoid of value.

At this time, Dr. Usui created the five principles of Reiki. He left the Beggars Quarter and began to teach throughout Japan. It was also at this time that the purpose of the symbols he had experienced in his vision became clear. He would use them to attune people so that they could take responsibility for their own well-being. By helping them amplify their energy, they could take a bigger step toward their own mastership. As the old dross was cleared away Usui began to train other teachers, young men who would join him in his travels. Shortly before his death, around the turn of the century, Usui charged one of his most devoted teachers, Dr. Chujiro Hayashi, a retired Naval officer, with the responsibility of carrying on the traditions of Reiki. Dr. Hayashi founded the first Reiki clinic in Tokyo.

In 1935, Hawaya Takata, a young Japanese-American woman from Hawaii appeared in Hayashi's clinic. She was very ill with a variety of organic disorders, and also lacking energy due to depression over the death of her husband a few years earlier. Having been on the verge of surgery while visiting her parents who had returned to Japan, she heard the voice of her deceased husband urging her emphatically to avoid the operation. After conferring to the doctor her reservations about the upcoming surgery, he recommended that she try the Reiki clinic, and it was there that she began to receive treatments, and was finally healed.

Takata was understandably impressed with Reiki and decided to learn it herself. Reiki had become a man's domain, and that meant hands-off to women. Takata was a typical determined "Gaijin" (alien) woman and did not give up easily. Her persistence ultimately paid off, and she was finally instructed in both First and Second Degree techniques. Later Takata returned to the U.S. and began her practice. In 1938, Dr. Hayashi and his daughter came to visit her. Soon after, Takata was initiated as a Master and the Hayashis returned to Japan.

Dr. Hayashi was a powerful mystic. He could sense that a war was coming with the U.S. and began to make preparations. Mrs. Takata sensed his concern and decided to return to Japan. Dr. Hayashi immediately warned her of the coming trouble. He already knew what the result of the war would be. He knew that Japan would be destroyed and that many of the men would die. He warned Mrs. Takata of the preparations she would need to make in order to protect Reiki. Not wanting to be drafted to participate in the violence of the coming war, Dr. Hayashi decided to make his transition. One day in the late 1930's, in full ceremonial dress, and amidst friends, Hayashi consciously left his body. Mrs. Takata stayed for a short time to help with his funeral arrangements, and soon returned to Hawaii, where she fortunately escaped the incarceration of Japanese-Americans during Would War II. In addition, this gutsy little lady pursued the teaching of Reiki in post-war America during the McCarthy era, a very closed-minded period of America's history.

In the 1970's Mrs. Takata began to train other Masters, and at her death in December of 1980, 21 had been trained. Today there are over 300 Reiki Masters teaching around the world.

My own goal as a Reiki Master is to assist each of my students to "fine tune" the vibratory level of his or her physical and etheric bodies, which in turn facilitates the development of higher consciousness. As more of us take the responsibility to raise our conscious awareness, the earth in turn will also be fine tuned to higher levels of Emanence.

All truths wait in all things,
They neither hasten their own delivery nor resist it,
They do not need the obstetric forceps of the surgeon,
The insignificant is as big to me as any,
What is less or more than a touch?

Logic and sermons never convince,
The damp of the night drives deeper into my soul,

Only what proves itself to every man and woman is so,
Only what nobody denies is so.

Walt Whitman

CHAPTER 3

How is Reiki different from other healing modalities?

The key to Reiki is its simplicity. Where other forms of therapy may demand months and years of training for the practitioner, Reiki can be taught in a weekend. To a person who is still very attached to the intellect as a means of learning, and is conditioned that learning takes time, Reiki can be disconcerting. The real difference is in the attunement process which puts Reiki in the category of energy work. Reiki is a process of empowerment, something which western culture has had little acquaintance with since the Age of Reason. After having been through the attunement process, most nurses, doctors, massage therapists, and people well-acquainted with the touch and feel of the human body, notice immediate increases in the amount of energy or the feeling of heat emanating from their hands when doing treatments. Thus people with prior experience of the body usually receive immediate feedback of the change which occurs as a result of the attunements, not to mention the sensations which sometimes occur during the actual attunements. Others with less experience or sensitivity need time and practice doing treatments to learn to perceive the changes immediately. Actually most people do, it is simply that those with too many preconceived notions need to learn how to listen to the body, because a successful treatment requires a listening process. The extensive amount of experiential time I allot my students for practicing treatments seems to provide enough chance for feedback and verification that there are indeed different sensations being experienced by the "healer", if not as strongly initially by the practitioner. In

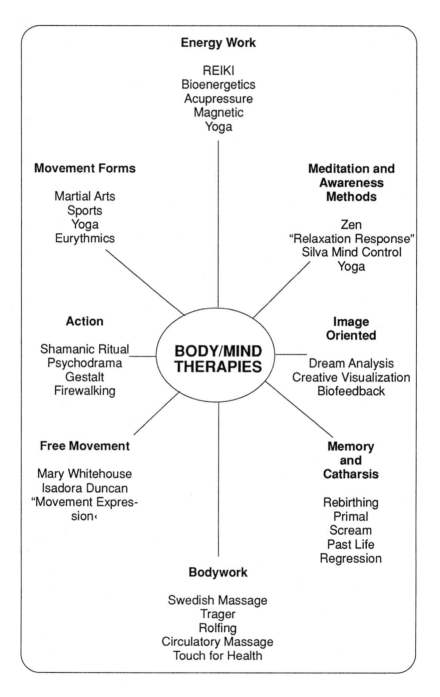

Energy Work

REIKI
Bioenergetics
Acupressure
Magnetic
Yoga

Movement Forms

Martial Arts
Sports
Yoga
Eurythmics

**Meditation and
Awareness
Methods**

Zen
"Relaxation Response"
Silva Mind Control
Yoga

Action

Shamanic Ritual
Psychodrama
Gestalt
Firewalking

**BODY/MIND
THERAPIES**

**Image
Oriented**

Dream Analysis
Creative Visualization
Biofeedback

Free Movement

Mary Whitehouse
Isadora Duncan
"Movement Expres-
sion‹

**Memory
and
Catharsis**

Rebirthing
Primal
Scream
Past Life
Regression

Bodywork

Swedish Massage
Trager
Rolfing
Circulatory Massage
Touch for Health

addition, I lead my students through a series of exercises to help them sensitize to the body.

My own personal experience as a massage therapist aboard a cruise ship years ago helped me to notice immediately the large increases of heat after only five minutes at the beginning of a Reiki treatment, compared to the minimal heat generated by giving 10 full massage sessions in a row! Naturally, I was impressed. Having been trained in a variety of bodywork techniques, but being primarily interested in deep tissue work, Reiki came as quite a surprise. I was of the mind set that it was necessary to do deep work to bring about really profound changes in the mind/body structure. It came as quite a surprise when some of my massage clients, whom I had begun to introduce to Reiki, along with their regular massages, began to ask me about that "interesting energy work" I had added to their treatments. Unexpected reports of vivid dreams, old pains disappearing, and creative spurts from artist friends began rolling in.

There were other interesting differences in this fascinating energy work that really struck my attention: Normally when a massage therapist is working on a client, and especially during deep tissue release work, it is necessary to keep the knees unlocked or slightly bent, similar to a Tai Chi stance. This is because the therapist acts as a grounding rod to the client. For example: If I am helping you release a large knot in your neck or shoulder, as I guide your breathing and you consciously release the lactic acid from the muscle, as long as my hands are on the knot, the negative energy being released runs into my hand, down my arm, and out of my feet into the ground. If ever I keep my knees stiff or locked during this process, your energy runs down my arm and body, does an abrupt u-turn at my knees, and returns to the exact spot in my body which is being released in yours.

It all sounds very esoteric when you are first learning about the movement of energy in the body, but it only takes a few unconscious moments to learn the truth of this process. It was quite a surprise to find that with Reiki this is not a problem or concern.

As I mentioned in the first chapter, Reiki is drawn by the healer through the open channel of the practitioner. The practitioner never absorbs energy from the healer, as the energy is always "outward bound" with the exception of what may be deposited and stored on the solar plexus – an added benefit. The healee, on the other hand, draws Reiki through a clear channel and thus does not absorb any of the personal energy of the practitioner/healer.

I have described some of the physical differences which make Reiki a very unique healing art. I would now like to share some of my own insights about Reiki from the aspect of my background in psychology. In other forms of energy work such as magnetic or mental healing, the practitioner must keep a constant focus on the sending of energy with no distraction from the client. In Reiki, once the initial intention to treat has been completed and the hands have been placed on the body, the energy will then be drawn of its own accord with no further intense focus from the practitioner needed. Thus if for some reason the client starts to "process" some old memories and emotions and feels the need to share, you can actually hold a conversation and continue to treat at the same time. Although this is an added benefit, I always discourage my students from initiating any talk, because most times the client tends to process at a level beyond words, and talking would be a great interference in the process. This I feel brings up an important aspect from a therapeutic standpoint. Many times, in my own past experience as a psychological counselor, the same people seemed to return time and time again with a different form of one basic problem. Sometimes it seemed that the more they would dwell on it verbally, the more it became "ingrained in the brain". Instead of releasing the problem, it just accelerated the problem. Of course, a good psychologist or counselor is trained to help turn negative ideas into positive ideas, and help the person release the pattern. With Reiki, much of the verbal release is unnecessary. During and shortly after a treatment, and especially throughout the 21 day cleansing period, after receiving either of the three degrees, people have a tendency to feel emotion bubbling to the surface. Sometimes direct memories are connected, but often only the emotion is released without the excess problem of intellectual attachment to a "story", which, in the long run, might more firmly ingrain the emotion – or block the mind/body structure from releasing it.

One suggestion I give my students is to acknowledge these emotions which sometimes appear unexpectedly, and to thank them (the emotions) for showing themselves and to let them go. By not suppressing them, but acknowledging them in a very conscious way, they seem to disappear quite quickly.

Another point about which some people need to be reminded, is the importance of letting emotion go. Many times, I've experienced a person, who after a long period of depression, finally moves to a stage where anger begins to be released. As anger is a higher vibratory energy than depression, the person may develop a tendency to enjoy the expression of anger without then moving on to a higher level of expression. Anger can be very seductive, because all of the drama involved really stimulates the ego to a high pitch. Anger is a result of feeling out of control. It is a result of failing to realize and take responsibility for all that we have created in our lives. It is so important to understand that you are only receiving what you at some time have put out – the Divine law of cause and effect. Life is your mirror. Thank that which comes along and release it, it doesn't have to continue. You are the creator. Realizing the importance of taking responsibility for all that you create in your life is indeed one of the keys of Reiki. Reiki doesn't end after the First Degree class. Each person must take responsibility to continue self-treatments. You are indeed your own master. Only you determine your rate of progress, by your level of commitment to yourself. The exhilaration which comes after each lesson is completed makes it all worthwhile.

From the above, we can see some of the unique aspects of Reiki. Like other therapies, it seeks to help each individual find balance and harmony in the Body, Mind, and Spirit. Reiki is truly a gift to yourself – when you participate in a Reiki class you are

acknowledging on some level: "I am ready to empower myself."
The power to co-create is your birthright. With that power comes
the privilege of greater responsibility, and a greater sense of unity
with your earth family.

Life is a balancing act.
to lose awareness of where
you are at anytime
is to risk falling off the
tightwire of life.

nari

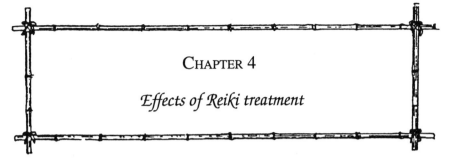

CHAPTER 4

Effects of Reiki treatment

Reiki affects each individual in a very personal way. The results of every treatment are determined by the needs (sometimes not always obvious) of the person being treated. There are some common denominators which seem to result in most treatments, and are listed on the chart of the previous page.

The format of a Reiki treatment will vary somewhat with each practitioner, however the primary focus will be on both any painful or "troublesome" areas of the body, and the endocrine system (refer to the diagram at the end of this chapter). Mrs. Takata taught a basic treatment pattern which covered all of these very important glandular systems, which in turn control the hormones of the body. To orthodox medicine, these glands are stimulated by neurotransmitters. The body communicates with the nervous system through the brain, which then stimulates the glands to release hormones that are needed for homeostasis. On the etheric level, each of the seven main chakras, or energy centers, corresponds to one of the endocrine glands (note the corresponding placement of the endocrine glands on the chakra chart in Chapter Ten). Thus, the endocrine system acts as a "transducer" of energy to the etheric energy centers, or chakras, and likewise the chakras act as „transducers" of energy back to the physical system through the endocrine glands. All levels are in some way interconnected.

To further explain this interconnection of the different systems, Dr. William A. Tiller, a Professor at Stanford in the Department of Material Science, and a research scientist for many years, offers a new theoretical model on the functioning of man. Up to the

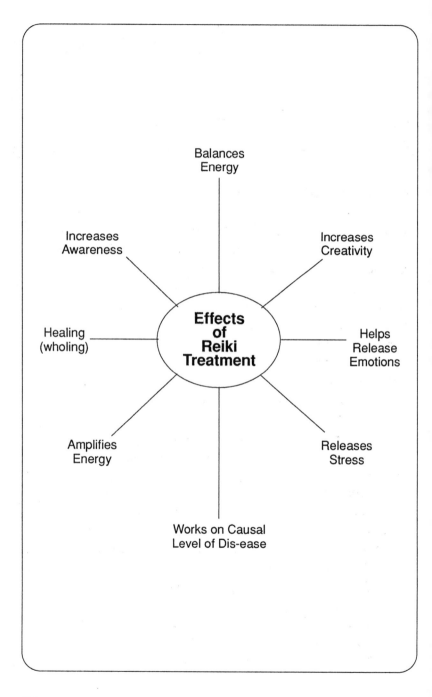

Balances
Energy

Increases
Awareness

Increases
Creativity

Healing
(wholing)

**Effects
of
Reiki
Treatment**

Helps
Release
Emotions

Amplifies
Energy

Releases
Stress

Works on Causal
Level of Dis-ease

present, most of the medicine, biology and agriculture community has viewed living organisms as operating via the following sequence of reactions:

function <– – –> structure <– – –> chemistry <– – –> electromagnetic energies, thus describing interactions only at certain levels.

Usually, flaws have been traced to structural defects that arose from chemical imbalance, with the "repair" procedure being an adjustment of the chemical environment (via drugs in man, or fertilizers in the case of agriculture). The dilemma that occurs is that both the organism (body or plant) and its threatening invaders adapt to the new chemical complex, in turn becoming less sensitive to it, so that an escalation of the potency must continue. The unnatural chemical content of the organism thus increases and begins to influence other levels of functioning, not only the one being "corrected", with often pernicious results. We can readily see the deadly effect in agriculture, where many grape pickers have died from high levels of toxic poisoning. In medicine, this type of procedure had resulted in many people suffering from iatrogenic (physician caused) disease. Fortunately, many physicians have become aware of this deadly problem and are taking a cue from Eastern medicine by adopting more preventative methods. On the electromagnetic energy level of the reaction scale, we already know the sometimes deleterious effects of x-rays.

Dr. Tiller questions the validity of the first equation. He sees the potential for physical and "nonphysical energy" procedures in the treatment of imbalance. Osteopathic physicians have had great success in treating human functions with direct physical manipulations. In addition he sees the serious reports of various types of nonphysical effects over the last two hundred years to suggest the naivete' of the first equation. Tiller proposes a reworking of the old theoretical model to a more multidimensional mode of substance. He proposes that the first equation be replaced

Endocrine System

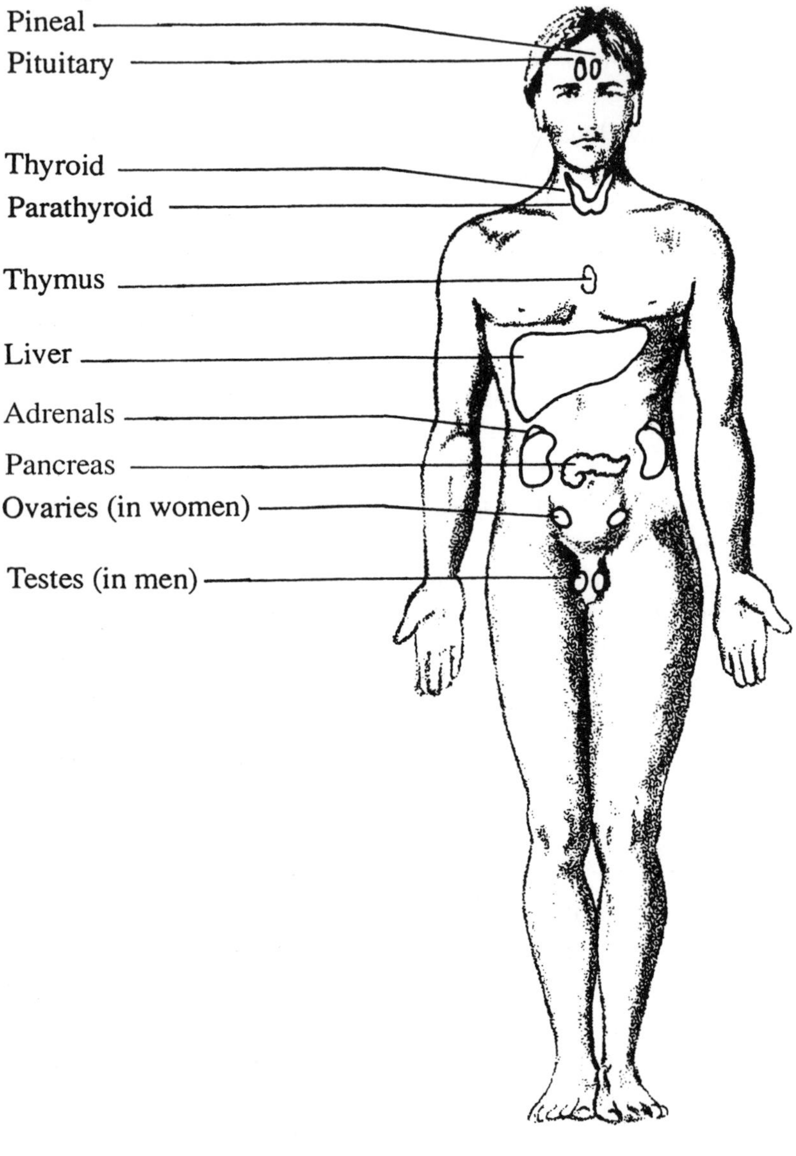

Pineal

Pituitary

Thyroid

Parathyroid

Thymus

Liver

Adrenals

Pancreas

Ovaries (in women)

Testes (in men)

by:

function <– – –> structure <– – –> chemistry <– – –> positive space-time energies (the physical body) <––––> negative space-time energies (the etheric body) <– – –> Mind <– – –> Spirit <– – –> Divine. He uses positive space-time energy to describe the physical body, and negative space-time energy the etheric body, in order to illustrate their kindred or coupled nature; as well as, the algebraic sign of their respective mass and energy states. To illustrate some of the link-ups in this expanded model, Tiller points out the mind/structure link in hypnosis, the mind/structure/function in Aikido, Zen or Yoga, mind/chemical and chemical/mind in psychiatry, in addition to many others. Tiller states:

> "The foregoing leads quite naturally to a perspective on healing, i.e., that pathology can develop at a number of levels and that healing is needed at all of them to restore the system to a state of harmony. The initial pathology begins at the level of Mind and propagates effects to both the negative space-time and the positive space-time levels."

Tiller then proposes that the best healing mode is to help the individual remove the pathology at the cause level and bring about the correction by a return to "right thinking". He states that the next best healing mode is to effect repair of the structure at the negative space-time level (etheric body). The next best level of healing is to effect repair of the structure at the positive space-time (physical body), which is practiced by medicine today.

As previously stated, Reiki practitioners have always recognized the "link-up" of the etheric and physical bodies through the connection of the chakras and endocrine system. In addition, Second Degree Reiki teaches the practitioner additional knowledge to help deal with the mental level of disease, where the causal factor is found. It is quite obvious to Reiki practitioners, as Tiller mentioned, that the causal level of disease rests with the mind. I personally would take this one step further and state that the causal level is due to the mind being out of synchronization

41

with the Spiritual or Divine aspects of man. Thus Reiki energy naturally works on the physical, etheric, and mental levels.

I encourage my students to use Louise Hay's book of affirmations, *Heal Your Body*, which deals specifically with individual dis-ease states. These affirmations help the healee recondition his or her mind, which in turn helps in the release of the causative factor. In addition, as I have mentioned before, Reiki helps each individual release energy blocks and the connected emotions, which in turn helps the release of the causal level of disease.

CHAPTER 5

The five Reiki Principles

Dr. Usui developed the five principles of Reiki shortly after he decided to leave the Beggars Quarter of Kyoto. It was at this time that he became aware of some important aspects of human nature. Usui had begun his healings with the hope of giving the beggars the opportunity to become reintegrated with society. When several of them tried and failed at shouldering the responsibilities of everyday life, he began to realize the importance of a person's participation in his own life healing process. A person needed to want and then ask for a change/healing to make a real difference in his life. If the help of others was involved, there should also be an exchange of energy. By just giving away healings, he had further impressed the beggar pattern in many of them. He saw that people need to give back for what they receive, in order to maintain a sense of balance.

Usui thus discovered two very important factors: one, that a person should ask for a healing. (It is not the job of any healer to try and help where healing is not wanted.) and two, that there should be an exchange of energy for the healer's time. (It is not right to keep a person feeling indebted for services rendered, thus the healee, by sharing energy in a variety of forms, frees himself of obligation.)

Dr. Usui also learned the importance of non-attachment to the results of his healings. It is possible that some of the beggars needed to live out their lives in the Beggars Quarter in order to learn certain lessons. Who are we to judge this as right or wrong? The same applies to disease – perhaps people "create" disease on a subconscious level to enable them to learn certain lessons, or perhaps, even to die. To a gifted healer, such as Usui was, to try to then interfere with a

43

"premature healing" might be a real transgression into a person's essential life process. It became very clear to Usui that it was not his job to use his incredible gift to "heal the world", but indeed, to show people how they might help themselves. It was at this time that he realized that people needed guidelines to help them grow in understanding, and to help them shoulder greater responsibility for their own life situations. He then understood why all of the great religions concentrated on the healing of the Spirit, as it seemed that the causal factor of disease lay in a rift between the Mind and Spirit. To change one's situation in life there had to be a change in attitude, as what you think, is what shall be. If indeed, all is mind, as is the first premise of Hermetic Science, then what we choose to project with our mind, is indeed what we will manifest on the physical level. To project only thoughts of love and gratitude is to create a life filled with love and abundance.

All of these concepts became clear to Dr. Usui after his years of experience in the Beggars Quarter. He had seen many people come and go, and had also seen many return to their old ways. Usui decided to seek out people who really wanted to transform themselves. Christ's maxim, to "not throw pearls before swine", became clear. One should not waste precious time and energy sharing information or energy with those who are not interested or prepared to receive. The five principles that Usui taught emanate naturally from a person in his or her proper flow. At the same time, trying to live the principles also helps put a person in that flow, because again, what you think is truly what you are.

Half the problem of getting
an answer
is being willing to listen
nari

The following are the five Reiki principles:

1.)
Just for today, I will live the attitude of gratitude.

To live in gratitude is to live in abundance. When we are constantly in the attitude of gratitude, feeling thankful not only for what we have received but for what we know and trust will constantly be provided, we begin to magnetically attract abundance. Our normal state is that of abundance. It is only our connection with the race mind consciousness (or collective unconscious) of lack, and our own conditioning, which keeps us from accepting that which is truly ours. One of the fundamental concepts at the root of the major philosophical and religious systems in ancient times, was that of all-sufficiency. It was taught that to understand one's self was to understand God, that by going deep within, one could transmute fear into love, ignorance into wisdom, and lack into abundance. In the Nag Hammadi texts, discovered in Egypt in 1945, which contain gospels older than those of the New Testament, Philip quotes Jesus as saying: "...what you see you shall become." In other words, if you focus on what you do not have, you will continue to be in lack. On the other hand, if you continue to be aware of the unlimited abundance all around you, and consistently feel the resulting gratitude, abundance will continue to be your state of affairs, and even increase. There is nothing lacking on this planet, it is the distribution system that has gone awry due to our illusions about lack, not to mention Man's greed, due again, to fear of lack, that has indeed kept us in lack.

To be in gratitude is to know at the core of your being that all is one, that separation is an illusion. Another important factor here is to be able to accept the abundance that is right fully yours. If you feel subconsciously "unworthy" of the riches and wealth of the Universe, you will block the flow of abundance to you. Many people now suffer from this consciousness of separation from *the* Absolute - that which embodies all that is. The long history of guilt of separation from the Absolute, keep even those people who seem to follow and live in accord with the laws of Universal Harmony, away from the true success and prosperity which is rightfully theirs. The causal factor must be sought in each individual. In most cases, the channels through which affluence and harmony normally flow are either undeveloped or paralysed. Universal Life Energy must then be used in order to give to those channels their natural functions. Once this connection is made, success and prosperity will be obtained. In the realm of the Absolute, every action, every cause, results in a perfect effect, which is complete success. The only reason that most people do not achieve it, is because they are not aligned with it, or are closed to it.

Hermetic Science teaches a simple way to align with the life force in your area, with the star exercise, where you stand for 3 - 5 minutes with your feet apart and arms and hands outstretched – left palm up and right palm down. The magnetic current in the surrounding area enters your left palm, and flows through the heart and solar plexus area, charging your entire body with the resulting surplus flowing out through the right hand. If done in the morning, you will feel energized. In the evening, a relaxing sensation will occur. For those who have been through the attunements of Reiki, it is recommended that you do self-treatments, which will give a much amplified version of this energy.

Once you have made contact with the Universal Life Energy and feel it flowing through the entire body, you should then focus your entire attention on feeling successful, and feeling prosperous and rich in all aspects of your life. The Life Energy will then amplify the channels of your inner self, and open them to the inflow of Universal Life Energy which, with its magnetic power, establishes the connection with all things you desire. The next step is to make a constructive effort to achieve your goals. Using only positive affirmations for success and prosperity will not bring them into existence. Affirmations must be sustained by Life Energy, the fundamental power of the Universe, in order to work. The resulting attraction, caused by the life force's magnetic current, along with constructive activity, will draw greater abundance into your life. Thus a bit of discipline is needed to change old patterns and create a prosperous flow. Making an effort to constantly bring your conscious awareness back to an attitude of gratitude, will in itself set up a magnetic attraction to Abundance. Self treatments will, in turn, help to clear away old subconscious patterns which might be blocking your flow of prosperity. Begin now to live in abundance, and just for today, live the attitude of gratitude.

Humanly - I seek the outward expressions of abundance sources of my good and welfare. Such error is to be corrected through progressions of lack and limitation until I realize that I do no-thing. Through the grace that is within All, outward forms of joyous abundance come into harmonious being effortlessly.

nari

2.)
Just for today, I will not worry

To worry is to forget that there is a divine or universal purpose in everything. If we are truly in tune with the guidance of our Higher-Selves, and live each day to the best of our ability, we are then aware that we have done everything in our power that we possibly can, and the rest is up to the Universal Life Force. Worry is a thought pattern which results from a feeling of separateness from the "I AM" consciousness (or Universal Wholeness). To worry about the past is futile – we must remember that each person (including ourselves) does the best that he can in each of life's situations, in accordance with the knowledge or wisdom he has at any given moment. We are all products of our conditioning and tend to react accordingly. If you regret a past action of yours, realize that you reacted according to your resources; then be thankful for the lesson and move on. At the same time, realize that all injustices done to you in the past were done by others as a result of their conditioning. We can only wish them well and hope that they too have learned from their actions.

To worry about the future is also futile. I have a saying that I live by: "Expect the best in life, and when you receive something that you didn't expect, know (trust) that it is the best for you in your present situation." Even if what occurs seems very negative at the time, it is only a lesson. Somehow, you helped create that situation, even if on a subconscious level, to learn. So feel gratitude that it has come to pass, and that you are free; then move on. Surrender to your Higher-Self, and try not to interfere with the Universal timing in life. Know that in your perfect flow there is a synchronicity of events. As long as you have completed your part in the scheme of things, all else will be taken care of. Worrying results from illogical and irrational patterns of thought, creating in turn more limitations and a further separation in consciousness. Surrender today to your Higher-Self's plan and release yourself from worry.

3.)
Just for today, I will not anger

Anger, in reality, is a totally unnecessary emotion. Like most inappropriate reactive emotions, it has its roots in the feeling of guilt from having separated ourselves from the Universal Consciousness. To anger is to desire control, which results from feeling out of control, indeed out of synchronization with our divine or universal life purpose. Many people have allowed their ego to direct their life course, at the same time ignoring the inner guidance which would otherwise lead them to a natural and harmonious flow. By allowing the ego to be effected by inappropriate desires and expectations, we suffer untold grief.

When our expectations get the best of us, and we become angry, because someone didn't live up to our needs and desires, we tend to forget that those we have drawn into our environment are only our mirrors. Every thought that we think sets up a cause, and the effect may come back when we least expect it. Truly, every situation is a mirror, a direct reflection of cause and effect, created by you. Those who happen to "press your buttons" or stimulate your weak points, are not really the cause of your anger. They are there to learn as well. You draw each other in a mutual need to complete certain lessons. Carlos Castaneda put it very well in showing appreciation for the "petty tyrants" in his life, because it is through them that we discover the weak points of our ego. By observing our reactions to others, we can determine what issues of attachment are still at work within our own psyches and begin to change negative patterns. Thus, when someone spurs you on to anger, try to stop the emotion, as Gurdjieff has suggested, in order to become more consciously aware of your reactions, and, in time, master your emotions. As you will discover with this exercise, it is impossible to stop anger in the middle of its expression, nor is it desirable to actually "stop" or suppress it. Indeed the whole purpose of the exercise, is that you begin to be aware of the roots of your anger. Such self-knowledge is an important first step. Also feel gratitude for having been given the opportunity to witness your weak points, as only growth can result.

Ultimately, I must point out that you should not feel guilty for experiencing anger. It has been programmed into us for so many generations, that it is difficult at first not to be triggered when we are "attacked" by the anger of others. In addition, we have long allowed our expectations to get the best of us, and tend to take things personally when things don't go our way. The hurt feelings which result cause us to lash out in anger. While attempting to "reprogram our old anger tapes", we must allow ourselves to release our emotions, and not hold anger in. We must feel our emotions fully. What we can do is tone down our reactions by expressing, in a calm way, how someone's negative statement makes us feel. If the other person persists in a loud way, it is wise to leave their vicinity and regain your power by not reacting. The best action to take, in the beginning of any episode, is not to react , but to emanate love. It is difficult to feel anger while you are smiling. Your smile may even trigger a "mirror effect" in the other person.

Finally, anger is a very disharmonious energy which creates disease in the body. It would be of great benefit to learn to transform this energy by dealing with it constructively. Just for today do not anger – be in the attitude of gratitude.

We create our
own dragons
nari

4.)
Just for today I will do my work honestly

Of great importance to a harmonious life flow is honesty in dealing with oneself. To be honest with oneself is to face the truth in all things. Many of us live in a fantasy world when it comes to perceiving reality. When we deny the truth about reality and are ultimately faced with truth, we may become severely disjointed. Sometimes the truth seems hard to deal with in our world, but if we really look deeply, examine our own behavior, and discover the purposes that various people and situations have in our lives, we will develop compassion for all.

To live in truth is to be aligned with your Higher-Self's purpose. Living in truth is also the simplest, least complex way to live. Truth brings clarity. When we face life honestly, we can more clearly see the lessons that we are here to learn, and complete them with much less effort. Living a life of illusion is much more complex. Denial then takes a center focus, and soon a web of falsehood may so thoroughly bind us, to "protect" us from the truth, that we may have difficulty finding our way out of the maze.

If you are honest with yourself, you will tend to project honesty onto others. It then becomes easy to "do unto others as you would have others do unto you". When you do your work honestly, you are being truthful to your Higher-Self. This truth is reinforced by love for yourself and others, which helps to create harmony in your life. So, live in truth vitalized by love, and just for today do your work honestly.

5.)
Just for today I will show love and respect
for every living being

Truly, we are all of one source. It is also clear that all forms of life are interdependent. The destructive changes that have occurred in recent times on the planet, (which have happened as a result of Man's insensitivity to the delicate ecological balance), have opened us up to this fact. In order to survive, we are discovering that we will have to drop our self-centered tendency to want to control nature, and learn to show love and respect for all life forms.

Through the study of physics, we now know that we are all a collective energy from the same source. There is truly no solid matter, only different levels of vibration. All forms of matter vibrate at different energy levels, yet they are all interconnected, because there are no solid barriers between them. Thus when we accept all of the various aspects of ourselves, it affects all others. Likewise, when we accept others, we too feel the reflection in ourselves. As a result, any positive energy, whether directed at ourselves or others, helps to heal the whole planet. Each person, animal, plant, and mineral is included in the whole. To show love and respect to all others is to love and respect ourselves and our mother earth.

The Principles of Reiki

Just for today I will live the attitude of gratitude

Just for today I will not worry

Just for today I will not anger

Just for today I will do my work honestly

*Just for today I will show love and
respect for every living thing*

CHAPTER 6

What are Attunements?

Attunements are the very core of the Usui method of natural healing. Reiki is the Japanese word for Universal Life Force Energy, something which we all have as our birthright. Anyone can lay hands on another person and transmit magnetic life force energy. What makes Usui's system unique is the attunement process, which may be described as a series of initiations wherein a Reiki Master, using a very ancient "Tibetan technology", transmits energy to the student in an amplified state. The energy acts in such a way that it creates an open channel for cosmic energy to flow in from the top of the student's head, through the upper energy centers and out through the hands, for use in future treatments. In addition, the vibratory rate of the body is amplified, triggering a 21 day cleansing period, which occurs as a result of negative patterns and blocks being sloughed off due to the quickening of a person's energy pattern.

The attunements are very precise and can only be transmitted by a Reiki Master who has been trained in Dr. Usui's method. There are two main schools of Reiki. One is headed by Phyllis Lei Furumoto, who is Mrs. Takata's granddaughter, and is called the Reiki Alliance. Several of the original 20 Reiki Masters trained by Takata are members of this group. The other organization, called the American International Reiki Association (A.I.R.A.), is headed by Dr. Barbara Weber Ray, and for the past couple of years, has used the term "The Radiance technique" for describing Reiki. Reiki Masters from either group are fully qualified to give the attunements, it is simply a matter of finding one that you resonate with. There are also a few, like myself, who are indirect products of both organizations. For example, my own Reiki Master/Teacher learned First and Second Degree through A.I.R.A. and Third Degree through a Reiki Master connected to the Reiki Alliance. Many Reiki Masters give introductory lectures in different cities. It is wise to attend one or two of these lectures to find the teacher who suits your needs. All are qualified Masters, but like teachers in any field, each has his or her unique focus, so it is good to find one with whom you feel a mutual bond or resonance.

One thing I like to point out to my students is that the attunements affect each person differently, depending on your vibratory level when you first receive them. In other words, if you have spent time doing work to expand your conscious awareness, and have reached a high vibratory level, the attunements will provide a very quick "quantum leap" to an even higher level. To someone just beginning consciousness work, there is also a "quantum leap", but the expansion of energy will be relative to the level that you start out with. The wonderful thing about Reiki is that, even after the "Quantum leap" which is caused by the attunements, you can still continue to increase your vibratory level and healing capacity by treating yourself daily and treating others whenever possible.

First Degree attunements are focused mainly on opening up the physical body so that it can then accept (channel) greater quantities of life force energy. The four attunements of First Degree raise the vibratory rate of the four energy centers of the upper part of the body, which are also known as Chakras. The first initiation attunes both the heart and the thymus while also attuning the heart chakra on the etheric level. The second attunement affects the thyroid gland, and on an etheric level, helps to open up the throat chakra, which is our communication center. The third initiation affects both the third eye, which corresponds to the pituitary gland (our center of higher consciousness and intuition), and the hypothalamus, which affects the the body's mood and temperature. The fourth initiation further opens the crown chakra, our connecting link with spiritual consciousness, and it's corresponding physical partner, the pineal gland. This final attunement completes the process by sealing the channel open, so that you can maintain the accelerated ability to channel the Reiki energy for the rest of your life. Thus it is essential to complete all four attunements to keep the Reiki channel open throughout your entire lifetime. Once you are attuned to the Reiki energy, you can never lose it. Even if you don't use it for a period of years, the moment you decide to use it, it will be there for you.

The Second Degree attunement process provides a "quantum leap" in vibratory level, at least four times greater than First Degree. The three symbols which are taught in Second Degree, to be used for sending absentee healings, also become activated at this point. Second Degree has great emphasis on adjusting the etheric body, rather than the physical body, which is the primary focus of First Degree. In addition, the third eye or sixth chakra is greatly affected, which often heightens the intuitive abilities of the student. Soon after the Second Degree attunements, and especially during the 21 day cleanse process, people often feel a considerable amount of energy in their root chakras, because their survival and sexual centers become very stimulated,which amplifies what Hindus call Kundalini energy. I often teach my students techniques for transmuting some of this energy into another form, to be used for stimulating the intuitive and spiritual centers to even greater conscious awareness.

The Third Degree attunement is used to initiate a Master. This attunement again amplifies the vibratory level and activates the Master symbol so it may be used to help others empower themselves. This is an important point, because it is essential for people to realize that it is their choice to receive an attunement. A Reiki Master holds no lordly power over his or her students. A Reiki Master is simply someone who has chosen to accept greater responsibility for their life by acknowledging that he or she is indeed the Master of his or her destiny. As co-creator with the Absolute, he openly accepts the effects of causes which he has created. By accepting this responsibility, the Reiki Master is empowered to use specific "ancient Tibetan technology" to help others further empower themselves. The attunement process of Reiki is really exceptional in that it enables you to get a sense of your true essence. We tend to sense our essence at times in our lives when we are in a heightened state of awareness. Reiki provides the boost to help experience that sense of awareness, and with a daily practice of self-treatments, that awareness can continue to grow. When you decide to complete the Reiki attunement process, you can look forward to an amplification of your conscious awareness, and a cleansing period to release old patterns. When you begin the attunement process, you take a positive step toward acknowledging your own mastership.

The infinite wind is sweeping my heart, body, and soul, bringing me the breath of a new beginning.

nari

Chapter 7

The First Degree class

One of the first questions that is asked by First Degree students is why there are different degrees in Reiki. During Usui's time, students would travel with him, slowly becoming initiated in the various levels of energy until they too could become teachers. In modern times, the division of attunements into degrees has made it easier to disseminate the various stages of energy amplification. Before completing each successive step, it is good to allow each student an adequate period of time to adjust to the higher vibratory level, and master the uses of the specific level. During the First Degree class, the student receives a permanent attunement to the Reiki energy, which occurs through four initiations. These initiations help to adjust the vibratory level of the recipient so that more energy can be channeled through the body. Adjustments also occur on the etheric level.

Reiki is a very simple technique when it comes to application. There is no intellectual process involved in learning Reiki, thus even children can learn it in the normal two-day class duration. First Degree is usually taught in four three-hour sessions. Initially the student is given the history and related background of Reiki, as well as the basic hand positions for self-treatment. The first two attunements are then given and each person begins to do a self-treatment. It is at this point that people discern the difference between before the attunement, and after the attunement, by the increase in either heat, tingling or pulsations, which begin to be felt in the hands.

The second session begins with exercises for developing kinesthetic sensitivity, after which the positions are given for laying hands on another. The remaining time is then spent on group treatments. The students then begin to feel the differences in energy drawn by each individual. Each student also receives an opportunity to experience a treatment from the group.

The third session begins with the final two attunements of the First Degree. Later there is discussion about the different feelings and experiences that the participants have with the attunements. I again encourage them, at this point, to keep a 21 day journal (refer to Chapter 5), as it is good to take note of the changes that occur, so that one can refer to them later for a greater sense of verification that the Reiki process does indeed facilitate cleansing and healing. I also encourage students to begin a self-remembering exercise each evening before going to sleep. It is so important in today's world that we each take responsibility to become more consciously aware.

Many people are not aware that in truth we are all in a type of hypnotic state or trance 24 hours a day. Hypnosis itself is only a tool to help focus the mind on one thing at a time. Indeed, most people experience the physical effect of loss of peripheral vision, while under hypnosis. They become truly one-sighted. During most of our normal waking hours, we are "hypnotized" by our conditioning. We experience a broader view in our normal lives than under induced hypnosis, but our focus is on old patterns of behavior. Here is a common example: In our daily jobs we are familiar with the personalities of our co-workers and tend to have standard topics of conversation for each person. We just plug our brains into each situation and play out a variation of an old scenario which has proven itself to work in the past. Thus most of us, most of the time, are not really experiencing life, we are reacting to life by plugging into old patterns of response. When Christ said that we need to "become as little children", he meant that we need to look at life as fresh and new each day. We need to learn again to experience life as it truly happens, without allowing preconceived notions or old patterns of response, which can often cause us to misinterpret the truth in many of life's situations, to

60

take over. To "become as a child" is a real challenge for most adults. It takes a great deal of conscious effort and discipline to break free of our old patterns. There must be a willingness to review one's actions each day, and see what could have been done better. What old habits need to be broken? Actually you will find that some patterns of behavior, such as good manners, are quite positive. What we can add to these positive patterns, to make them even more effective, is our conscious awareness. In other words, when you say "Hi" to the passerby on the street, don't just mumble it out of habit. Look the person in the eye and connect. You will feel so much more alive, and will help the other person to feel the same way. When you walk down a crowded street, consciously send love out to those around you – it will make a difference. When you make a conscious effort to "wake up", others around you will tend to pick it up by osmosis. The wave of gratitude will flow through you, and with practice staying consciously aware, will begin to take less effort.

To help keep yourself in the flow, it is beneficial to do a nightly self-evaluation. Review your day mentally and think back to how you reacted to each person and situation. What was appropriate and what could have been changed? What do you remember most clearly? You will find that the memories in life, which you recall so clearly, are from circumstances which occurred when you had a flash of conscious awareness. This exercise will help you to become aware of your behavior. With practice, you will begin to "see yourself watching yourself." Also with practice, you will begin to see yourself catch yourself before giving an old inappropriate response in a new situation.

While you do this self-remembering exercise, it is very appropriate to give yourself a Reiki treatment. This will help you to further release old buried patterns of inappropriate behavior, and help rebalance your mental energies. In addition, you may feel yourself processing old emotions beginning to release them, as many behavior patterns tend to also be connected to past emotional reactions.

Another issue that I discuss in the First Degree class is that of helping people deal with a healing crisis. To begin with, whenever starting treatments on someone, it is recommended that there be a commitment from the healee to receive a minimum of three treatments in succession, over a three day period, if possible. There is often a "lag time" of approximately three days for energy to be transmuted from the physical body to the etheric body, and vice-versa. It is ideal to continue successive treatments during this period. As a result, if you are working on a person with an acute illness, they may experience more pain in the first two or three days of treatment, due to the acceleration of healing energy. The pain then seems to dissipate quickly on the third day. As a result, it is sometimes good to warn the patient that he might experience the illness more intensely at first, but that it will lessen.

When you are working on a person with a chronic illness, or one that has been active for a long time (such as arthritis), you will find that Reiki usually brings immediate relief. When treatments are continued on chronic illnesses, the patient will usually feel steady improvement for quite some time. In this type of case, if there is to be a healing crisis at all, it will usually occur several weeks after treatment. This is because the toxins, which caused the illness in the first place, are slowly released until the point when they only have one final "stronghold" in the body. It seems that the last toxins or vestiges of a problem are the hardest to remove. Sometimes, when a person gets to this stage (called Physical Chemicalization), he will experience the symptoms of the illness more intensely than ever before. It is at this time that you must reassure the patient that the symptoms are a good sign of final release of the toxins. Additional treatments should be added at this time, to speed the release of toxins. It is my suggestion not to warn people with chronic illnesses about the symptoms of healing crisis, because you may project a response in them that might not otherwise occur. If it does occur however, you are forewarned and can reassure them that it is a very normal reaction, and help dissipate their fears. Again, in case of an acute illness, it is good to warn the patient that they may experience Physical Chemicalization or sensations that occur as a result of a rapid physical response to the illness, as this occurs very often.

In any serious acute crisis, a person should be encouraged to see a qualified physician. Your treatments will then help to accelerate the healing as the healee draws only the energy needed to promote quick recovery. In the case of a chronic illness, the healee will most likely have already visited a physician. Your treatments will help to release toxins which have probably built up over a long period of time.

There is no definitive timetable for the release of acute or chronic illnesses with Reiki. Each person is unique in the way that they react to treatments. Each person truly heals himself. Reiki channels act only as vessels through which healees draw the energy they need to create balance on all levels of their beings. It is not appropriate for us to place attachments on the results of our work, or to make any judgements, as each person accepts the amount of energy appropriate to his or her needs, and the results of the healing are not always directly visible. We must always keep in mind that there are often secondary benefits to having a disease, and a person may not be ready to be healed on the physical level.

During the fourth session of the class, we begin with each student giving and receiving a complete one hour Reiki treatment with a partner. Treating one person's whole body helps the student begin to discern between the differences in heat which are drawn in different areas of a body. Each person has different needs, and will draw different amounts of energy in different areas accordingly. The student then learns to give more attention to areas of the body which are drawing more energy. To complete the class, we again proceed with group treatments until each person has had a turn being treated. Then we have a final question and answer session. First Degree certificates are then awarded and people are encouraged to continue meeting in groups to share treatments. Each class that I have taught has been a wonderful experience, as every individual is special and brings their unique energy into the group. So much personal growth and group camaraderie develop during the class, that many times it it difficult to end the class at the end of the weekend. The boost that we all receive, with the amplification of our energies, really helps us to awaken to the awe of knowing who we really are. When the time is right for you to join a First Degree class, you will know.

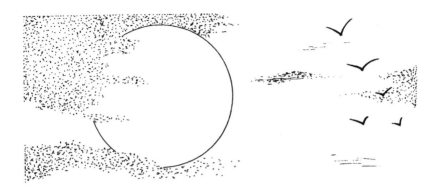

I am the wind, sea, and sail
I am the ship for any gale
I am the sky, cloud-filled blue
I am it all, strong and true
I am setting off to far new lands
I am it all, godself in man.

Nari

CHAPTER 8

The 21 Day cleanse process

After the attunement process in each of the three degrees, the student will undergo a 21 day cleanse process. Due to the raised vibratory rate of the physical and etheric bodies, old dense negative energy is forced "to the surface", and is released. As we know from the study of physics, solid matter does not really exist. Everything is composed of energy, thus everything has a vibration. Even rocks and minerals are made of energy, they simply have a lower rate of vibration. In a similar fashion, negative blocks and emotional patterns, which are stored in our physical and etheric bodies, have a lower vibratory rate than the thought waves or pockets of energy that we create when we are thinking loving and positive thoughts. Thus as we increase our vibratory rate, through steady persistence at whichever spiritual discipline we choose to study, we begin to notice how much easier it is to maintain a positive flow, due to the snowball effect.

When we receive a series of Reiki attunements, the sudden amplification of vibratory rate acts as a trigger to set off an accelerated loosening of negative, dense energy within our systems, which cannot resonate with the finer vibrations created by the attunements. Since your vibration is adjusted so quickly, a reaction takes place which allows old stored-up emotions and memories to be released, as is appropriate for further growth. Although the change is sudden, it takes time for the adjustments to become effective. It takes approximately three days for the energy to move through each of the seven main chakras. Although the opening of the Reiki channel occurs between the heart center and the crown chakra, the centers in the lower part of the body are equally important and go through a corresponding adjustment in vibratory rate.

Some of the typical outward signs you may notice in your life as a result of this cleansing process, include various dreams, "strange feelings", emotional changes, physical changes such as detoxification, and an old habit or favorite food, which loses its importance in your life. These are just a few of the possible symptoms of the change which occurs at different levels of the physical and etheric bodies. Some reactions may seem unpleasant at first, as the negative energy is released, but by just saying "yes" to each experience, accepting it and not attaching a great deal of concern, each one will simply pass away.

I often suggest to my students that they keep a journal during this process to record the changes which occur. In addition, it is helpful to give your self the simple suggestion, "I will remember my dreams the first thing in the morning", and then leave your journal at your bedside so it is there when you first wake up. You will find that after a week of persisting with this suggestion, that your dream retention increases dramatically. Dreams are a wonderful tool to help us tune in with our subconscious. Although they may seem nonsensical or unclear at first, with persistence, a pattern will begin to emerge. It is good also, at this time, to develop a habit of giving yourself Reiki treatments before you fall asleep at night, and first thing after you wake up in the morning (after writing down your dreams). If you continue to treat yourself after the initial cleanse process is completed, you will help the growth process to continue, and further refinement of your energy will occur. As you release old undesired feelings and concepts, you will begin to feel the attitude of gratitude flow naturally in your life process, which will in turn create a greater level of abundance in all areas of your life.

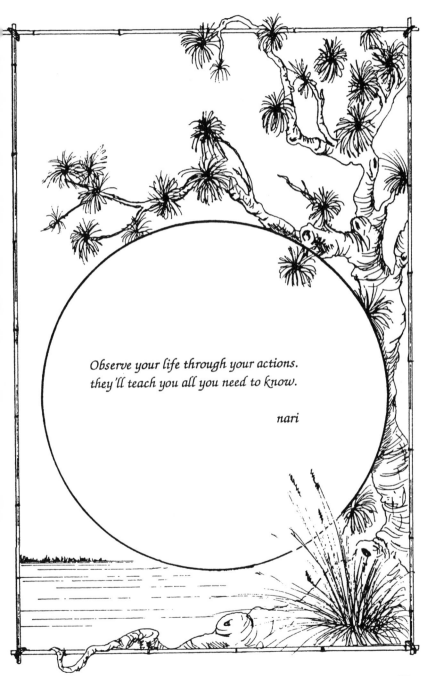

Observe your life through your actions.
they'll teach you all you need to know.

nari

CHAPTER 9

The Second Degree class

The Second Degree class provides the participant with the opportunity to attune to higher levels of the Reiki energy. The initiations of Second Degree also attune a person to the power keys or symbols, which are used at this level to perform absentee and a stronger form of mental/emotional healing. As Second Degree activates another level of energy (an amplification of vibratory level in both the physical and etheric bodies), you will again experience a 21 day cleanse period, similar to the one experienced in connection with First Degree, as your body and different energy centers adjust to an even finer level of vibration. Additional techniques for your own growth and further development are also taught at this level.

First Degree attunements focus on elevating the energy of the physical body, so that it may channel more intense healing energy, whereas Second Degree attunements work more directly on the etheric (bioplasmic) body and tend to stimulate development of the intuitive center which is located at the pituitary gland. Hermetic Science recognizes the pituitary gland to be the telepathic apparatus of the human body. Hindus call it the Eye of Shiva, and in the West it is known as the third eye. The pituitary gland is infinitely delicate and sensitive, and acts as a sending and receiving station for mental vibrations. After receiving Second Degree attunements, it seems that the normal spherical waves of thought which emanate from this center, and normally dissipate easily, are sharpened and become more easily focused in both their incoming and outgoing functions. Thus, in time, it becomes easier for a Second Degree student to receive information on an intuitive level.

The development of intuition is vital in our age, because it serves as the mouthpiece of our Higher Selves. By listening and reacting to the voice of our Higher Selves, we will find that we are on our proper life path and in a harmonious flow with those around us. Life then takes on a pleasant rhythm and all of our activities become synchronized. The Higher Self truly knows everything, as it is not limited by time or space, and it does not need reason or logic to aid in its activities. Intuition knows because it simultaneously embraces cause and effect, the past, present and future. If we choose to follow intuition, we will find that we will end up with positive results, even if it sometimes seems to argue with the conclusions of the intellect. In order to further develop intuition, we must learn to differentiate between the voice of desires placed in our minds by mass consciousness and those placed by our Higher Selves. One simple way to discriminate between the two is to notice the very different feelings that are evoked by inappropriate desires, and by those of the Higher Self. When the voice of intuition speaks to one, a sense of peace and harmony is evoked, even in a seemingly disharmonious situation, while inappropriate desires tend to bring on an unsettled feeling. Thus it is better to listen to the voice of peace and wisdom, which brings a sense of harmony, than to heed the aggressive clamor of inappropriate desires, which only lead to ultimate dissatisfaction. The more you listen to your intuition, the more it develops. With practice, it becomes easier to follow the guidance of one's Higher Self, and increase one's confidence and wisdom. Second Degree gives a powerful boost to the development of this sixth sense, and continued self-treatments using the Reiki keys helps to increase one's intuition to an even greater level.

During the Second Degree class, you are taught three keys which help to focus your mind so that it can send the Reiki energy beyond time and space. These keys unlock the Reiki power for those who have received the Second Degree initiations. There is nothing magical about the keys. They serve only as focus points for the practitioner's mind, to enable the Reiki energy to be channeled over long distances, and to amplify it for mental/emotional healing. The basis for the keys is found in age old universal laws that concern the transference of energy through the use of the mind. Because most thoughts are sent out like rays of light darting from a central point, they tend to lose much of their original force as they spread out – much like the waves created by throwing a pebble into a still pond. In contrast, to send a thought over a great distance, it must be concentrated, made one-pointed. The Reiki keys are the answer that Dr. Usui found, which immediately enables a Second Degree practitioner to "send" the Reiki energy across time and space. To say that the energy is sent is, in a sense, a misnomer. Even in Second Degree the energy is drawn by the healee, not sent by the "healer". With the keys, the practitioner actually forms a "bridge" between himself and the healee, so that the energy can then be drawn as needed.

The Second Degree class is usually taught on a weekend over three evenings. On the first evening, the keys and most of the intellectual information are passed on, in addition to the actual attunements. On the second evening, much of the time is spent learning to apply the keys and a special technique that promotes healing on the mental level. The third evening is focused primarily on absentee healing. A variety of possibilities for using the keys are discussed, and the student is encouraged to further explore these possibilities.

The mental/emotional healing technique helps to release the negative conditioning from past experiences. Often in life, we have reacted to certain circumstances in a negative way. When similar circumstances arise, instead of approaching them with an open mind, we usually react in what has become a "pattern", even if such a reaction is inappropriate. "Negative" experiences themselves also tend to program us in unconscious ways. Sometimes we find ourselves reacting to situations without any forethought. One of the Reiki keys, when used properly, helps to release these old patterned responses.

Much of the time, physical illness is caused by the mind being out of synchronization with the spirit. Insight into the causes of certain illnesses can be found in Louise Hay's book *Heal Your Body,* and in Chapter 16 of this book, which explains how the various parts of the body harbor certain types of emotions, and can thus cause corresponding illnesses. All of this information can be used along with the mental healing technique. This ultimately helps the receiver of the treatment come into closer contact with his Higher Self. The Second Degree student can also use this technique on him or herself, which helps to develop clearer intuitive faculties, as the old patterns are cleared away. There is much movement and growth which takes place as a result of taking the Second Degree Reiki class. The student should be prepared to experience change on several different levels. The changes which come, result in the empowerment of the student. With the empowerment comes greater responsibility, which is rewarded with greater healing power. Second Degree provides an opportunity to become consciously aware at a higher level. To take a Second Degree class is to "wake up" to further dimensions of one's Higher Self. The voice of intuition becomes truly alive, and a greater sense of wholeness, peace and harmony results.

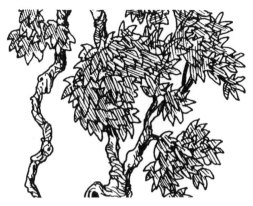

Human beings, in developing within themselves that
Divine Ray of Intuition, will manifest Wisdom,
will become six-pointed stars, stars of wisdom,
and will bring about the Dawn of the New Day,
The Day of Peace, of Harmony and Power.

Eugene Fersen

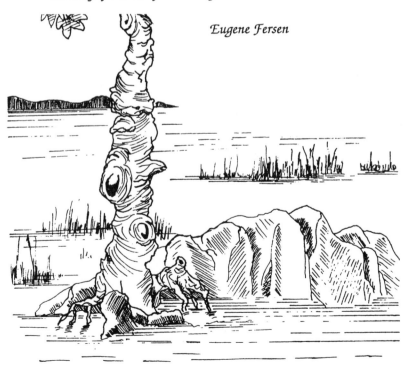

CHAPTER 10

Extra tools to use with Reiki

The following tools are not connected directly to Reiki. Many students, after completing Second Degree, receive very clear intuitive messages to guide them in the healing process. Mrs. Takata herself added a variety of procedures to her treatments, which were not passed down from Usui. Each one of us has our own unique talents, and should feel comfortable about experimenting and even expanding our own repertoire of healing methods. Because Reiki treatments do not require a constant focus of attention on the channeling of energy to the healee, the healer is left with an opportunity to observe and concentrate his thought processes elsewhere. While Reiki, in and of itself, is a complete healing modality, you may choose to investigate some of the following methods in combination with a Reiki treatment:

a) Removing Energy Blocks

Occasionally, while giving treatments, you may notice that a particular area of the body seems to draw very little or no energy and perhaps even feels cold to the touch. When you are quite sure that you are feeling an energy block, and that your hands don't feel cool because they are drawing enough energy to feel hot in comparison to the patient's body temperature, you may choose to utilize the following technique: After having laid your hands on a very cool area of the body for five to ten minutes, without any sensation of energy being drawn in a quicker fashion, you may intuitively sense that an energy block is present. In order to remove it, you can scoop the energy into a tight compressed ball at the surface of the skin, grasp it with your left hand, and lift it away from the body. Sever it with your right hand by making a slicing motion next to the surface of the skin, and then lift the right hand to the left using it to surround the left in white light, and let the ball of energy go. When you return your hands to the body, you will generally feel a definite increase in the flow of energy, because the person is now free to draw and accept more Reiki.

One thing that I must point out about this procedure is that it is possible to do it entirely in the mind's eye. In other words, there are times when the personality or belief system of the patient is such that to move the hands as I have described, would seem like "mumbo-jumbo." On the other hand, there are times when certain people would benefit by visually seeing you extract the energy as verification that something negative has indeed been removed. As Albert Schweitzer stated:

"The witch doctor succeeds for the same reason all (doctors) succeed: each patient carries his own doctor inside him. They come to us not knowing the truth. We are at best when we give the doctor who resides within each patient a chance to go to work."

Thus it is a healer's priority to find out just what might trigger his or her patient's belief system.

While involved in research in the field of parapsychological healing methods, I discovered the aforementioned technique for removing energy blocks, while studying with a Mexican Spiritualist healer. I also observed at that time that people are aware, on a subconscious level, of energy blocks in the body. Sometimes dramatizing the actual removal of these same blocks helps to convince the conscious mind of the healee that a change has indeed taken place, and thus accelerates the healing. Often the person will experience the movement of energy in the body or heat during the procedure. Reiki itself is very powerful and will gradually diffuse most energy blocks in time; however, using such a conscious process as described above helps to remove blocks more rapidly.

Energy blocks themselves are created in a variety of ways. For the most part, they are a result of stored emotions which have not been able to be expressed. Chapter Sixteen gives an in-depth look at the various causes of emotional blocks, and in particular, which types of emotions are stored in specific areas of the body. Another cause of energy blocks is due to negative thoughts, which when a person becomes obsessed with them, seem to take on an energy or life force of their own. These may eventually attach themselves to the body in a large mass. Theosophists call these thought forms, which have taken on a life of their own, elementals.

The average person doesn't realize that our thoughts are indeed very powerful. All of our thoughts amass in the etheric or energy body of the earth, which is why it is so important that we become consciously aware individuals. Thoughts which pass through us quickly do not generally take on a life force of their own, and are soon dissipated. However, if a person becomes obsessed with a negative idea over a period of time, the force of these thoughts will create actual "little beings" called elementals, which will in turn help perpetuate the same thoughts. Long standing family and national feuds are powerful examples of the life force in elementals. On the other hand, positive thoughts which are repeated over and over also create a life force of their own, and will perpetuate themselves. It is very important for people to understand this phenomenon, because at the present time, with the powerful love energy entering the earth to create healing, many people are experiencing large awakenings which are affecting their intuitive faculties. Some are even developing the ability to see elementals, and begin to think they are losing their mind, due to the lack of cultural references to explain such occurrences. Certain countries, such as Brazil and England, who are fortunately more open to these phenomena than most, have a variety of organizations who deal in such matters and can educate people. This is quite necessary, because it is important to note that often people who are institutionalized for "seeing things" and labeled as schizophrenic are only uneducated psychics.

There is great fear in large areas of Western society about psychic abilities. This is largely due to the centuries of witch trials, in which millions of people were burned and tortured, that resulted in the demise of the intuitive faculty, and the development of logic and rationalization which reached its height under the reign of such thinkers as Descartes. In our world, rationalization and logic have come to dominate thinking, but it is plain to see that it does not solve all of our problems. Today we see a blend occurring as the intellect begins to take its proper place beside the intuitive faculty and is relegated to its proper place as a tool of the mind. Even the most successful businessmen are those who follow their intuition rather than rationalization and logic, as is seems in the many books in the business section of bookstores for developing intuition. As we begin to develop greater ability in the intuitive realm, some of the very ancient and very normal human psychic abilities are returning. We are all naturally telepathic. It is clear that even animals have these abilities; that indeed they think in pictures as has been shown by certain psychics reading the minds of sick animals, to help aid veterinarians in diagnosing their illnesses. If animals have these abilities, then why shouldn't humans? More and more of my students are developing greater intuitive abilities, especially after receiving Second Degree Reiki. People must realize that these are God-given abilities.

When people experience psychic abilities in a negative form, they need to look inside for the causal factor. If a psychic experiences attacking "monsters", it is usually the experience of one's own negative elementals or thought forms. These can be released when seen visually by canceling them, to transmute the energy. Truly, there is no evil, only ignorance. Even such things as "possession" can only occur if the person believes on a subconscious level that someone else can have power over him or her. Anyone who would try to possess another also does so out of ignorance, as cause will bring the effect back to them. For centuries we have given much of our power away to the governments and religions. It is these institutions that really possess us.

Now it is time to take back the responsibility where it lies - in ourselves. We must begin to choose our governments and our religions consciously, and not blindly follow our parents as they did their parents before them. Following the blind keeps the same emotional blocks and denial alive through each generation. We must break the chains of ignorance and mass hypnosis by removing the blocks that are located throughout our bodies, which were placed there as a result of the denial of who we truly are - co-creators with the universal life essence. Truly we are beings of light, and the more we recognize this, the higher our collective vibration will become. It all evolves around true conscious awareness of who you are. Reiki can help this process by bringing back energy and balance to areas of the body which have been long denied the nurturing and healing qualities of the life force energy. Take the time to listen to your body, and feel the areas which may be blocked. Daily self-treatments, especially using the Second Degree mental healing technique, will help to release outmoded patterns of behavior. You may experience long withheld emotions coming up, in addition to interesting dreams. As you get a sense of the cause of the block or denial, using your knowledge of the area of the body from which it comes (see Chapter 16), you can begin to formulate affirmations to permanently eradicate any negative thought forms. Louise Hay's book, *Heal Your Body,* gives an excellent selection of affirmations for individual medical problems, and *Reiki - Universal Life Energy* by Bodo Baginski and Shalila Sharamon has an excellent section devoted to the esoteric cause of physical illness. Using these tools and your own intuitive abilities, you will begin to formulate the appropriate program of healing for yourself.

b) Using Color and Sound

There are many books available which discuss the powerful healing effects of color. Dr. Joyce Nelson of San Diego, California, completed a research project which tested the effects of various colors on people whose eyes were exposed to colored lights. During the experiment, the subjects were monitored by a polygraph machine and tested for galvanic skin response. When the subjects viewed a violet light, several of them eluded to drops in their pulse rates. On the other end of the scale, males were more susceptible to a rise in pulse rate, when viewing red, than females. During her research, she also discovered many of the healing properties of color. She uses this information, in conjunction with her knowledge of crystals, to teach classes in natural healing. Dr. Bara Fischer of Santa Fe, New Mexico, offers seminars introducing the Darius Dinshah method of color therapy. This entails shining one of twelve different shades of color on a client, depending on the symptom. The following list illustrates the qualities of each color, and their effects on the body:

Red: Energizes the nervous system and stimulates the senses. Activates the circulatory system. Helps to heal infections, x-ray damage, and ultra-violet burns.

Orange: Helps to strengthen lungs and bronchial tubes. Stimulates the thyroid and stomach. Relieves cramps and helps to build bones.

Yellow: Stimulates the lymphatic system, motor and sensory nerves, digestion, and increases hormone production.

Lemon: Nourishes the body and brain, helps to clear lungs, stimulates over all body repair.

Green: Balances the physical body and cerebrum, stimulates pituitary and acts as a germicide.

Turquoise: Repairs acute problems, and heals burned skin.

Blue: Acts as a sedative, lowers fever, releaves inflammations, itching and irritations. Also stimulates the pineal gland.

Indigo: Sedative. Stimulates parathyroid, shrinks abscesses and tumors, and acts as an emotional depressant.

Violet: Activates spleen and white blood cells, helps to reduce fevers, and relaxes muscles.

Purple: Lowers body temperature, heart rate, and blood pressure. Also acts as a kidney depressant, and controls lung hemorrhages.

Magenta: Balances emotions, adjusts blood pressure to perfect balance, and stimulates adrenals and kidneys.

Scarlet: Stimulates adrenals and kidneys, emotions and reproductive organs, and raises blood pressure.

I encourage my students to explore the use of color, not only in healing, but in everyday dress. Sometimes, while guiding a person through a Reiki/Rebirthing session (see Chapter 11), I encourage the recipient to wear the color which corresponds to the chakra or energy center where emotional release is needed. In addition, I have found Jon Monroe's audio color tapes to be of great help in emotional release work. Jon has made recordings of the twelve sounds or tones which match the twelve colors of Darias Dinshah's vibrational color scale. The vibrations of color actually correspond to the different vibrations of certain musical notes. Playing the corresponding chakra color of an emotionally blocked area of the body, during release work, helps to promote further healing.

c) Crystals

Quartz Crystal has become very popular in recent years as a tool which helps to amplify and direct the natural energies of the healer. With the quantum leap taking place in man's consciousness, some of what is thought to be ancient Atlantean crystal technology is now coming to light. In addition to the exploration of crystal healing methods, which are being conducted by many individuals, traditional science has also discovered the powerful properties of the crystalline structure. In recent years, science has begun to utilize crystal technology for solar power, communications, and information storage. The piezo-electric effect, which occurs when crystals are placed under pressure, and as a result, emit measurable electrical voltage, is one property which is now being utilized. In other words, by mechanically squeezing a quartz crystal, it begins to emit electrons. Conversely, applying an electrical current to a crystal, causes mechanical movement. The regularity at which the mechanical movement occurs is quite precise, which is the reason why quartz crystals are so useful in keeping time.

Crystals occur in nature over many areas of the planet, and in recent years science has developed the technology to grow them synthetically. A crystal is a geometrically formed fused mineral, sugar or substance, whose molecules or atoms are arranged in a repeating pattern, which gives the external shape a symmetrical appearance. The stable geometrical/mathematical orderliness which crystals maintain with extreme precision is also a clue to their usefulness as a programming tool. Their capacity to form and hold a specific energy matrix and transduce information between the subtle levels or planes of existence is another key to their usefulness as a healing tool.

In Chapter Four, the interconnection of the different bodily systems, and the extreme versatility of the Reiki energy, which enables it to penetrate all of the various systems, were discussed. Whereas Reiki energy penetrates the physical and etheric bodies simultaneously, as well as, penetrating the mental level where the causal factor of disease lies, crystals seem to work primarily on the subtle energetic bodies. As has been previously mentioned, disruptive patterns in the etheric body can often be seen by clairvoyants and registered by sensitive instruments before they manifest at the physical level in the form of disease. Herein lies the inherent usefulness of crystals, which is to amplify and focus energy directly at specific areas of blockage in the etheric system. If disease is already manifest in the physical system, the positive changes that crystals help to make on the etheric level will eventually also effect correction on the physical level. Thus crystals are a great help in removing energy blocks and negative thought forms on the subtle energetic level, but they will not necessarily be able to release a long ingrained mental or emotional pattern which lies at the causal level of disease. From the above information it can be seen that crystals provide us with a powerful tool to amplify and direct healing energy, but they cannot prevent the healee from recreating the negative thought form which created the illness in the first place.

Reiki, on the contrary, provides a powerful method for working on the causal level of dis-ease. There are also many ways that crystals may be used with Reiki to promote further healing. While Second Degree Reiki offers a complete system for absentee healing, the First Degree student can program a crystal with Reiki by holding it between the hands and charging it with Reiki energy. You may then loan or give it to someone who needs healing so that they may treat themselves or carry it on their body. Crystals can be charged with a healing thought form which is sent out over a distance by holding the crystal and visualizing the energy being received by the healee. As crystals operate at the level of magneto electric frequencies (subtle energy levels), the mind-directed energies of the sender are amplified and simultaneously transmitted from a distance to the healee. The Second Degree student can further program a crystal with the special mental healing technique to further amplify the energies needed to effect change on the causal level. Such a process using the Second Degree level helps to further activate the crystal to higher levels of vibratory frequency. Randall and Vicki Baer, the authors of several books on crystal technology, point out a distinct difference between charging and activating crystals.

Crystal charging is the renewal of a crystal's vibrational charge, whereas activation increases it's overall charge capacity. My own experience has shown that First Degree Reiki charges a crystal, and Second Degree tends to actually activate a crystal by increasing its overall charge capacity.

One other interesting factor that I would like to point out, which helps to explain the wonderful resonance between living beings and quartz crystals, is the fact that human beings are living crystals. Biological science is beginning to realize that several substances and membranes within the human body seem to function as liquid crystals. Marcel Vogel, a well known researcher at IBM for over twenty-six years, has found that by cutting a quartz crystal in a very precise manner, it can be tuned vibrationally to the exact frequency of water. Since the human body is made up largely of water, it is not surprising that we resonate so well with quartz crystals when they are used for healing purposes.

In August of 1988, I had the great pleasure to meet Dr. Igor Smirnoff and his wife Irena, two researchers who had recently immigrated from the Soviet Union. Both have been involved for years in the water birthing process, and Dr. Smirnoff has actually invented a special crystal device to program the birth water with dolphin and whale sounds. The babies are put in a special swimming program immediately after birth, and it seems that their intuitive capabilities become highly developed. Within a few short weeks, the infants can sleep comfortably on their sides floating on top of the water. The infants are actually able to stand on their feet only six weeks after delivery, and when tested floating in a glass tank, in total darkness, they can find their mothers standing at either side of the tank. The phenomenal abilities and sensitivity that these children exhibit seen to show some of the important links between the programming capabilities of crystals, water, and human beings.

The following information is a very brief guide to help you understand the basics of crystal use. For more in depth information, you may refer to the recommended reading list.

Choosing a Crystal

The main factor in choosing a crystal is to find one which resonates with your energy field. Just as people have different energy patterns, crystals also have their own unique vibrations. The color, size, shape, and type are all important factors in crystal selection, along with the intended use. Your best guide is your intuition, and your own sensitivity to the subtle energy field coming from the crystal. Dr. Joyce Nelson, the author of *Crystal Gypsies' Guide To: The Metaphysical Properties Of Color*, and an expert in color and gem therapy, recommends the following exercise to help develop sensitivity to subtle energies:

Step one: Rub your palms together briskly for about one minute.

Step two: Move your hands (palms facing each other) slowly apart until they are around six inches apart, then slowly move them toward each other until they almost touch. Continue doing this as you try to feel any tingling sensations, heat changes, or any other subtle energy change in your hands. Once you have developed this sensitivity, try moving your hand over the top of a group of crystals, to feel a similar energy.

Clearing and Cleansing Crystals

After purchasing a crystal, or receiving one as a gift, it is wise to clear it, as quartz crystal tends to absorb any vibrations which are (or have been) in its close vicinity. Crystals tend to absorb and store the energy and thought patterns of people who have held them or been in close contact with them. Crystals which are worn or used daily should be cleansed on a regular basis (at least once a week). Those which are generally kept in a harmonious environment need only periodic cleansings. Some of the various methods for clearing crystals are, soaking them in a salt water solution for at least twenty-four hours, placing and covering them in dry sea salt for at least twenty-four hours, cleansing them with running water, and also by blowing on each of their facets while visualizing them becoming clean and pure.

Charging Crystals

In order to renew the vibrational charge of a crystal, several methods may be used. You can put the crystal in the center of a crystal gridwork or under a pyramid for a number of hours. Surrounding crystals with color gels and projecting light is one way to charge them with the different vibratory rates of color. Also, leaving crystals in a highly energized point on the earth, such as in a vortex area or one with a low geomagnetic pressure, will help to give a charge. Finally, Reiki is a very powerful tool for charging crystals. Charging can be accomplished by any Reiki practitioner who holds a crystal between their hands, with the intention of charging it, and then focusing on the purpose for which they wish to use the it.

Activating Crystals

As mentioned earlier, the activation of a crystal involves expanding its overall energy capacity so that it may accept a greater charge. Randall and Vicki Baer, in *The Crystal Connection*, recommend exposing a crystal to high and very low temperatures to induce activation. However, the temperature changes must be gradual to prevent any cracking of the crystal. Exposing them to extreme weather conditions such as lightning storms, blizzards, are also mentioned, along with the use of Tesla coils, electrostatic generators, and even more elaborate crystal gridworks. Second Degree Reiki can also be applied to increase crystal capacity.

Crystal Programming

Just as science now uses crystal technology to store memory in computers, the individual can learn to program quartz crystals for many different purposes. Programming is essentially the process of storing specific energy and thought patterns in a crystal. The following two examples of crystal programming are taken from *Crystal Gypsies Guide to Crystals* by Dr. Joyce Nelson:

Healing:
Your crystal can be programmed for specific health problems. Visualize the person's health problem (or any other kind of problem) getting better, feel the healing energy flowing into the crystal, visualize the problem completly healed. Be as detailed as possible. After the programming process, you can give the person a treatment by holding the crystal over their body and guide the energy where you want it with your mind. Visualize the energy flowing from you through the crystal and into the person's body. You can also give or loan the crystal to the person and have them treat themself or just carry it with them. After a few treatments it is advisable to cleanse and reprogram the crystal.

Color Programming:
Every color has a certain vibrational quality that can be used for numerous purposes. Color can be used to induce changes in personality, emotions, states of mind and physical disorders. The color for the change that you desire is programmed into the crystal and used in the same manner as above. See the *"Crystal Gypsies Guide to the Metaphysical Properties of Color"* for further specifics on what colors to use. Colored plastic gels can be put around the crystal and placed in front of a light source (sunlight, light box, in front of a lamp, etc.) to enhance the programming process.

Crystals are neutral objects which emit energy, and extend and amplify their programs in a coherent, highly concentrated form. As previously mentioned, programming is the process of storing specific energy and thought patterns so that they may then be transmitted into objects of people at will. It is important to note that anyone choosing to work with crystals should exercise responsibility, because, although they may be used for mind to mind communication, their higher purpose, as Marcel Vogel has pointed out, is in the service of humanity for the removal of pain and suffering. For those who are acquainted with the history of Atlantis, whether you take it as fact or myth, it stands as a powerful example of the need to take caution and exercise increased individual and collective responsibility for the higher levels of technology which are currently being developed. Crystals can be programmed as powerful tools to help the individual promote further self-transformation. When used with Reiki, the possibilities are as limitless as the human mind.

d) Chakra Balancing

The direct link between the endocrine system and the seven main chakras was discussed in Chapter four. It was established that the Usui System of Natural Healing (Reiki), has always recognized the "link-up" of the etheric and physical bodies through the connection between chakras and the endocrine glands. Chakra is a Sanskrit word which means wheel. The term is appropriate, as the chakras appear to be spiraling disks of light to someone with clairvoyant abilities. The location of the chakras in the etheric or energy body corresponds directly to the placement of the endocrine glands in the physical body. The etheric body is an energy body of very fine vibration which totally envelops the physical body. Both are interconnected by currents of energy. The etheric body absorbs finer levels of energy from the environment, and transduces this energy through the chakras into the physical body via the endocrine glands. The endocrine system controls the hormone balance in the body, which has a powerful effect on a person's mood and emotions. Thus, it can be gathered from above, that if the chakra system is out of balance, its counterpart, the endocrine system, is also out. If an imbalance somehow occurs first in the endocrine system, it too will put the chakra system out of balance, because energy moves back and forth between the two. Reiki energy is absorbed by both systems simultaneously, making it an excellent modality for creating balance in both the chakras and the endocrine glands. Because the Reiki practitioner feels the energy being drawn in greater amounts wherever it is needed in the body, there is little guess work involved in trying to find areas that are out of balance.

As can be seen by the accompanying diagram, not only are the endocrine glands effected by the chakras, but the surrounding organs and certain sections of the nervous system are as well. Each of the chakras also has a specific function which corresponds directly to certain types of emotions and factors in human development. Some of the different purposes associated with each chakra are listed on the diagram. If one of the chakras is out of balance, its associated function in the individual is also out of balance to some degree.

All of the chakras are of equal importance. This is necessary to note, as many people tend to focus solely on the development of the upper chakras because they are more "spiritually" connected. The fact of the matter is that everything is a manifestation of Spirit, and if one chakra is out of balance, they are all out of balance. The lower chakras tend to be more attuned to earthly energies, as can be seen by their connection to specific earth elements, and the upper chakras to more etheric or cosmic forms of energy. The heart, which is at the center of the body, is the meeting place of the two energies. It is the place where the two polarities, spirit and matter, meet in the expression of love. As heart is of the element air, it is truly the meeting place of heaven and earth. We need to focus a great deal of attention, at this time, on the development of the lower four chakras, as growth in these areas will help to ground us to our Mother Earth, and help in the healing of the planet. We must not forget that matter (earth), the female/mother polarity, needs just as much recognition and love as (heaven), the male/father polarity.

In order to balance the chakras and promote healing on all levels, full Reiki treatments are very much in order. If you desire a briefer technique, the following are also effective:

Standing Method: With the healee standing sideways, you place one hand a few inches in front of the lower belly and the other hand just a few inches away from the tip of the sacrum,

7) Crown Chakra (Sahasrara)
Endocrine system: Pituitary gland
Physical organs: upper brain
right eye
Function: connects us with
our spiritual self

5) Throat Chakra (Vishudda)
Endocrine system: Thyroid
Physical organs: throat
lungs
Function: communication
self-expression
clairaudience

3) Solar Plexus Chakra
(Mani pura)
Endocrine system: Adrenals
Physical organs: stomach, liver
gall bladder (digestive system)
Function: Power and wisdom
center
Element: Fire

1) Root Chakra (Muladhara)
Endocrine system: Suprarenal
Physical organs: kidneys,
bladder, spine
Function: survival issues
physical vitality, seat
of Kundalini, creative
expression, abundance
issues
Element: Earth

6) Third Eye Chakra (Ajna)
Endocrine system: Pineal gland
Physical organs: Autonomic nervous
system/hypothalamus
Function: Intuitive center
seat of will and
clairvoyance

4) Heart Chakra (Anahata)
Endocrine system: Thymus
Physical organs: heart, lungs
liver, circulatory system
Function: Love, compassion
Element: Air

2) Sacral or Splenic Chakra
(Svadhisthana)
Endocrine system: gonads
Physical organs: reproductive
organs
Function: center of sexual energy
- feeling/emotional
center
Element: Water

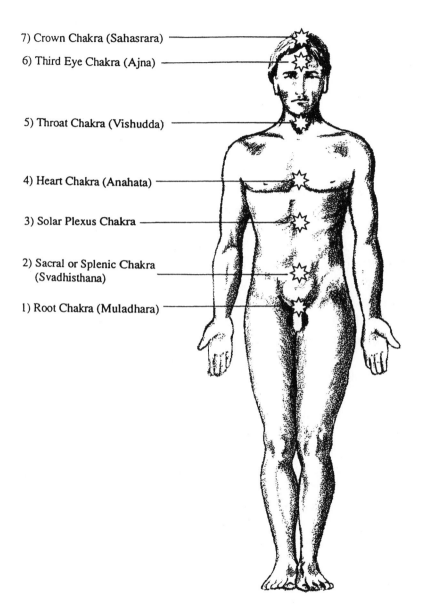

7) Crown Chakra (Sahasrara)

6) Third Eye Chakra (Ajna)

5) Throat Chakra (Vishudda)

4) Heart Chakra (Anahata)

3) Solar Plexus Chakra

2) Sacral or Splenic Chakra
   (Svadhisthana)

1) Root Chakra (Muladhara)

where the root chakra is located. Hold your hands there for two or three minutes until you feel a wave-like rise and fall of energy. Continue on up over each of the chakras for a period of two to three minutes, until you come to the crown chakra. Place your hands over the top of the head, leaving the fontanel uncovered. After several minutes, bring the hands down over the chakras, again ascending to the root chakra as you integrate the energies and close all of the centers.

Balancing heaven and earth: With the person laying supine, place one hand over the lower part (closest to the table) of the top of the head and place your other hand under the coccyx (tip of the spine). Wait until you feel a similar pulsation, tingling sensations, or heat, and then move one hand over the brow (third eye chakra) and one hand up to the belly (three finger widths below the navel). Again wait for similar sensations in both of your hands, or an intuitive sense that they are balanced. Next, place one hand gently over the throat and thyroid area (do not exert pressure on the wind pipe), and the other on the solar plexus. Wait to feel a sense of balance between the two chakras, and finally, place both hands over the heart center. When complete, gently and slowly raise your hands off of the body, while taking into consideration the sensitivity of it's auric field.

Be sure to engage your intuitive knowingness when balancing bodily energies. Feel free to connect different combinations of chakras, as each person has different imbalances, and might be aided in very different ways. Second Degree Reiki can also be used in this process by adding the symbols where appropriate.

Balancing the chakras ultimately creates balance in all of the systems of the body; therefore, it is appropriate to focus on these energy centers when performing Reiki treatments. The Endocrine system in the physical body will also benefit, and the corresponding rise in the vibratory rate of the body will promote greater conscious awareness.

e) Centering

In today's world, which is dominated by Western culture, most of us tend to identify with the intellect as being the center focus of the mind. Since the Age of Descartes, in the seventeenth century, when logic and rational thinking superceded intuition in importance, we also have tended to link the intellect very closely with the personality. Over hundreds of years, more than one million women and men were burnt at the stake as witches, almost entirely destroying the ancient culture of the wicca (wise) who had been the healers and medicine people of pre-Christian culture. Actually the irradication of intuitive/psychic abilities began during the dark ages while the religious sanctions against such abilities were promoted to gain further control over the masses by the ruling intellectuals, who used church politics as their weapon. The intellect began to take center stage to the point where today the church has been over shadowed by the hallowed halls of education. Universities, instead of the church, are now the primary conditioning agent for the mass mind/culture. The development of the intellect has reached its height and it has become apparent that it alone cannot provide all of the answers to the massive problems now facing humanity. To help meet the numerous challenges which lie ahead, we must recognize the intellect's true place as a tool, and not continue to identify with it as the essence of who we are. The next step that we must take is to redevelop our latent intuitive abilities.

Receiving the attunements of First and Second Degree Reiki helps to open up intuitive knowledge. Continued self-treatments also help to further development of this long dormant faculty.

During my Reiki classes, there is a very simple process that I like to teach my students, to help them focus their consciousness in their hara or feeling center of their bodies. When we are centered in the hara or chi center, as the Chinese call the emotional/sexual chakra (spleen chakra), the opposite polarity chakra located in the third eye also becomes balanced and opens up. By literally allowing the intellect to "step aside", and bringing the center of our attention (the focus of our conscious awareness), into the "belly" chakra, we begin to connect with our true feelings. Once we are centered in the hara, we naturally open up to the intuitive faculties located in the third eye chakra.

The process involved is quite simple: I ask the students to sit in a comfortable position either on the floor in lotus position with legs folded and back slightly forward, or in a chair (also leaning forward so that the spine is perfectly balanced and relaxed) with the ears over the shoulders and the shoulders over the hips. I then begin to lead them through the following visualization, which you may want to record on tape and play back to yourself:

Begin by taking nice long slow deep breaths. Inhale through the mouth and exhale through the nose. Good. Just keep on breathing – nice long slow, deep breaths. Begin now to visualize a beautiful golden glowing ball floating just above the top of your head. This ball is the golden glowing ball of your conscious awareness. Continue to breathe. See your breath expanding the golden glowing ball of your consciousness. Each time you exhale, the beautiful golden sparkling light of your consciousness emanates outward. Continue breathing nice long slow deep breaths. Take one more deep breath into the golden glowing ball of your consciousness. When you exhale, begin to see the golden glowing ball float gently down through the top of your head and begin to blend with the lovely purple glowing ball of the crown chakra. Take another deep breath into the now golden purple glowing light of your spiritual consciousness. Watch as it expands with your breath, filling with warmth and light, and as you begin to exhale, see the light emanate and sparkle outward, sending the beautiful light of your consciousness to those around you. Continue to take nice long slow deep breaths into the golden purple glowing ball. See it expand again with your breath, and then, as you exhale, see the beautiful sparkling light glowing, radiating outward. Continue to breathe long slow deep breaths. Inhaling slowly, and now as you begin to exhale, see the golden glowing ball gently separate from the purple center of your spiritual consciousness and float slowly downward to the center right behind your brow, the beautiful indigo glowing center of intuition – your third eye.

Notice the golden glowing ball as it melds and becomes one with the beautiful glowing ball of your intuitive knowingness. Continue to breathe. Take another deep breath into the now golden indigo glowing ball, filling it with the warmth and light of the breath, and then, as you exhale, see the beautiful golden indigo light permeating the air around you. Take a nice long slow deep breath into the the golden indigo glowing ball. Feel the breath filling it with the light of your intuitive consciousness and then sparkling and flowing out into the surrounding environment. Continue to breathe. Take one more nice long slow deep breath into the golden indigo glowing chakra. As you exhale, see the golden ball begin to gently separate from the indigo glowing chakra and descend slowly down toward the throat into the lovely light blue-turquoise glowing chakra. See the two become one, filling your communication center with the energy of your breath, and as you exhale, send the light and love from your communication center out toward those around you. Keep on breathing nice long slow deep breaths. As you inhale, see the golden turquoise ball fill with the light and energy of your breath. As you exhale, see the turquoise-golden light emanate and sparkle out toward those around you. Now begin to take one more nice long slow deep breath into the turquoise-golden glowing ball. As you exhale, see the golden ball again begin to separate and float slowly and gently down into the heart center, the lovely emerald glowing center of your heart. See the golden ball begin to merge with the lovely emerald green ball, filling your heart with the consciousness of your love. Continue breathing as you inhale. Feel the breath fill your heart with the light and energy of love, and then slowly, as you begin to exhale, see the beautiful emerald-gold light sparkling and radiating the energy of your love to all of those around you. See it continuing out in waves, washing over the planet filling it with love, and then, as you inhale again, feel the energy of love returning with your breath as it fills you and expands you with the emerald-golden glowing light of the heart center. Take one more long deep breath into the emerald-golden glowing ball, again filling it with the light of love, and as you exhale, begin to see the golden glowing ball of your consciousness begin to separate and float slowly down into the solar plexus – your center of power and wisdom. See the golden light merge and become one with the brilliant yellow glowing ball of the solar plexus right between the rib cage. Continue to take nice long slow deep breaths. See your breath expanding the now golden-yellow glowing ball with the energy of your wisdom and power center, filling it with the power of love.

As you exhale, see the light sparkling and sending out its rays of power to those around you. Take another deep breath, again filling the golden-yellow center with the energy of your breath, and as you exhale, feel the light and warmth of your power and wisdom radiating outward and filling each person with the empowerment of love. Take one more nice long slow deep breath into the golden-yellow chakra, and then, as you exhale, see the golden ball slowly begin to separate and float gently down into the lovely orange chakra, three finger widths below the navel, filling the ki or chi center with the golden light of your consciousness. With each warm breath, feel your belly filling with the golden-orange light of your emotional /sexual center, and as you exhale, feel the emotions of love sparkle their lovely golden-orange light to all around you. Continue to breathe nice long slow deep breaths, filling the belly with the emotions of love, and again sending the golden-orange light outward to those around you. Just keep on breathing into the belly, filling it with the consciousness of your love, feel the warm glow of the orange-golden light as your consciousness rests in your center. Feel the peace and tranquility. Continue to breathe. Take one more long slow deep breath into the hara, and as you exhale, see the golden light begin to slip away and again float gently downward toward the tip of the sacrum, down into the red root chakra. As the two merge and become one, feel the heat of the beautiful golden-red light begin to fill the entire pelvic area, filling it with the light of love and abundance. As you inhale, feel the golden-red light fill the pelvic area with the consciousness of love, transmuting all of the survival issues of this chakra with the energy of abundance. As you exhale, see the beautiful golden-red light sparkle and emanate toward those around you, sending your abundance outward in waves of light, and then, as you inhale, feel this light returning and filling you again with an overflowing of abundance. Just keep on breathing. With each breath you feel the energy of prosperity and abundance fill your entire body, starting in the root chakra and radiating out from there, continuing to fill the entire body. As you exhale, see the light and love of abundance flowing out around you. The next time you inhale, see the golden glowing ball gently separate from the red root chakra and float gently upward, back toward the hara, returning to the beautiful orange glowing light of your feeling center. As you exhale, see the orange and golden light become one. Continue to breathe nice long slow deep breaths into your center, feeling very tranquil and totally at peace. As you inhale, the orange-golden light fills your entire being with the emotion of love. As you exhale, feel all disruptive emotions fading away. Each time you inhale, you feel more fully grounded and at center, flooding your belly with the love energy of your breath. As you exhale again, see the orange-golden light of your love energy streaming out, overflowing with the abundance of your love; and then, with the in breath, flowing back to you with the same waves of love and abundance. Contemplate the peace and calm in your center, and the open channel this creates as you feel at one with all those around you, and with your environment.. As you relax in this calm center, slowly begin to open your eyes and again become aware of your environment.

The above exercise is designed to help you develop the feeling of being centered. As you move progressively through each chakra, you may occasionally feel resistance at specific chakras to the movement of your consciousness between them. If you feel blocked in any area as you follow this procedure, you can exhale several times in an abrupt and powerful manner to help "blow out" any clogged areas. Once you develop the feeling of being centered, you can shorten this exercise by exhaling two or three times, within seconds bringing the center of your consciousness quickly down into the belly, as you allow your intellect to step aside, and at the same time, put yourself into an alpha state, two of the benefits inherent in this centering exercise.

There has been much research done on psychic and spiritual healers which has shown that successful healers seem to work in an alpha state, which in turn, the healee seems to pick up by "osmosis" during the healing. One experiment that I encourage my students to try, is to walk into a crowded supermarket or department store alive with chatter and clamor, and take a few moments to become deeply centered. It is amazing how quickly the area around you grows calm and peaceful, and the conversation often recedes to a tranquil murmur. It is important to note that when this occurs, it is not you who is affecting the people, it is simply that the alpha state is absorbed automatically by those around us. In other words, when I am in alpha state, I act as a natural channel for this energy to be transmitted to others who are in my close vicinity. It is similar to the process that I used as a teenager to overcome grand mal seizures. I would "tune-in" to someone else's calm brain waves, and prevent an aura from becoming a full blown seizure. It seems that calm peaceful waves of energy tend to overcome the more static or disharmonious types of energy.

Taking the effort to center oneself on a daily basis is a sure way to maintain a more tranquil lifestyle. It not only will help to keep you in a state of emotional balance and health, but it may even permeate the energy fields of those around us without any real effort, and give them a boost of the same healing energy.

CHAPTER 11

Combining Reiki with other Healing Methods

Reiki blends well with a variety of different therapies. In the previous chapter, several tools and techniques were discussed which can be used in conjunction with Reiki treatments. One especially effective combination is used in conjunction with bodywork. Many massage therapists around the world combine Reiki treatments with Swedish, Circulatory, Sports, Shiatsu, Acupressure, Jin Shin, and Trigger Point massage, to name just a few. Other forms of bodywork, such as Rolfing, Emotional Point Release Work, and Polarity, are enhanced with Reiki. My own method for combining Reiki with bodywork is as follows:

Begin with the client lying face up. After doing a few minutes of neck massage, give a full scalp and deep facial massage. Next, perform all of the Reiki head positions and continue to cover the entire endocrine/chakra system giving extra attention where needed. Complete Reiki on the front of the body by treating the knees and feet. Covering the knees is very important as they hold fear of death, fear of death of the old self or ego, and fear of change (refer to Chapter 16). All of us are going through intense changes these days, so a large amount of energy is needed in this area. Feet have points that connect with the entire body which makes them a nice place to finish Reiki on the front portion of the body. Now return to the shoulders and apply oil. Now it is time to begin the massage on the front of the body. Once the legs and feet are finished, the client is asked to turn over and oil is again applied to the back of the legs and the feet, and then the back itself. Once the massage is complete, Reiki is applied to the entire back, which is followed by a final energy balancing technique on the spine.

The above is just one suggestion for combining Reiki and massage. Using your intuition as a guide, the possibilities for combining the various techniques are endless.

Also very important, is the combination of Reiki and allopathic medicine. Doctors, while palpating for tumors, can use Reiki to feel where the energy is being drawn, while at the same time, actually transmitting healing energy to their patients. It can also be used in the process of setting bones to diminish pain, and accelerate the healing process. Even pediatricians can use it in the care and handling of younger patients. More and more doctors are becoming interested in Reiki as they discover the myriad of ways that it can be used to enhance their treatments. Reiki also can help to improve the effectiveness of medication. Through the wonderful work of Dolores Krieger and Therapeutic Touch, the benefits of hands on healing have gained great acceptance in the medical field. With the amplified energy of Reiki, hands-on healing takes on a new dimension. Many nurses are being drawn to Reiki as they search for alternative healing methods which provide more personal contact, as well as a regenerative tool to use with their patients. Newborns, as well as, children and adults in intensive care units, benefit greatly from the treatments. Patients are also comforted by the soothing touch and energy provided by Reiki.

Naturopathic, Ayurvedic, and Homeopathic treatments are also enhanced with Reiki. Charging remedies with Reiki is a powerful tool for accelerating healing energy. Another powerful healing method used in combination with Reiki is fasting.

Therapeutic fasting is one of the oldest methods used throughout the ages to cure a myriad of dis-ease states, such as arthritis, asthma, skin problems, high blood pressure, digestive disorders, and kidney and liver diseases. Most diseases in man are self-induced through overeating, poor diet, and lack of exercise. Lethargy and overindulging in rich foods is a sure path to autointoxication. Disease then results when glandular activity and metabolic rate slow down, and the eliminative organs decrease in efficiency due to the steady build up of toxic deposits in the cells and tissues of the body. For example, rheumatoid arthritis is a result of uric acid crystals and mineral compounds which have collected in the joints and soft tissues. High blood pressure, along with stress, is a result of metabolic wastes which have been deposited in the arteries and small blood capillaries, resulting in a restriction in the blood flow. Fasting is a very powerful method for clearing all of these waste materials out of the system.

On the third day of a fast, autolysis begins to occur. After 72 hours without food, the body starts to digest its own waste materials. The first to be digested are always unnecessary toxins which are stored in the body, such as cysts, tumors, and excess mineral buildups. These are followed by the digestion of excess fatty tissue. It is also after the third day that the initial discomforts of feeling hungry, and possible dizziness or weakness all disappear. In Scandinavia, doctors who follow the biological route for curing their patients, use fasts anywhere from seven to sixty days in duration, with truly amazing results. If a patient is very weak or sick to begin with, they will be put on a healthy diet to build up strength, and later, begin the fasting procedure.

There are different types of fasts. Some are pure water fasts, and others combine fruit juices and vegetable broth. One even combines lemon juice, maple syrup and cayenne pepper, diluted in water. The key to any fast is to use only fresh fruits and vegetables. Using a juicer to make the appropriate drink just before you imbibe it is the ideal, in order to benefit from the raw live enzymes. One of the most popular cancer cures developed in the 20's and 30's, initially to cure tuberculosis, and later cancer, in the Max Gerson therapy, which is based on the premise that raw live foods act to cleanse and naturally strengthen the immune system of the body. Albert Schweitzer was a great advocate of Gerson's as his own wife was cured by this therapy.

During a fast, it is important to not only drink plenty of liquid, but it is also important to give yourself a couple of enemas each day to make sure that the bowels are kept clear of toxic materials. After three days of fasting, there is not always enough fecal matter to sustain parastaltic action, however, the toxins do still build up in the intestines, thus it is important to keep yourself flushed out to avoid autotoxicity. For those who are interested in fasting, it is suggested that you consult a wholistically oriented physician if you are trying it for the first time. There are also several books listed with more detailed plans for fasting, the proper way to come off of a fast, and other very pertinent information.

Reiki is a powerful tool to use with fasting, as it helps to alleviate any of the symptoms which might occur in the first three days. Also, it amplifies the life force energy in the body, which helps to boost the immune system, and speed up the process of elimination. For those pursuing a wholistic oriented biological cure, fasting, used in combination with Reiki, will provide a very powerful alternative.

Whereas fasting provides a very effective means for cleansing the physical body and eliminating years of toxic buildup, there may be times in life when we seek to clear out old and inappropriate negative emotional patterns, in order to create a more positive approach to life. The healing of the emotional body is just as important as healing the physical body. As stress and tension become stored in the body, and begin to mold its form over the years (see Chapter 16), the personality becomes molded as well. We tend to develop negative reactive habit patterns when we subject ourselves to constant emotional stress. To help release these patterns, which extend all the way back to the birth trauma, a technique called Rebirthing or "Conscious Breathing" has been used for over fifteen years. The original founder, Leonard Orr, began the development of Rebirthing in the early 1970's. Many sessions are completed in jacuzzis heated to body temperature, in order to effect a womb-like environment. A relaxed, rhythmic breathing is employed with each inhalation and exhalation, connected in one long unbroken chain. The breath is focused in the lungs or chest, rather than the diaphragm, and it is appropriate to breathe out of either the nose or mouth. The primary goal of the breathing is to move energy through the body. During the rebirthing process, it is common to feel tingling and vibrating sensations throughout the entire body. Many people experience a stiffening of the hands due to the release of long accumulated tensions, and to resistance to the energy flowing throughout the body. This is usually a signpost that a great deal of sadness is coming up and needs to be released. These symptoms come and go very quickly as the breathing pattern is continued. As each thought form is turned from negative to positive, with the help of a rebirther, much healing takes place. It is recommended that several sessions are carried out until you experience what Orr calls the Breath Release. This occurs when you re-experience your first breath. It evokes a powerful healing as the damage done at birth to the breathing pattern is healed, and your habit of improper breathing begins to disappear.

Another development in conscious breathing is the tendency in some people to regress back to past life memories. What is important to note is that whether we have lived before or not, these memories of past lives do exist. There are a variety of explanations, however, what is important is that these "stories" act as powerful tools to help one release long buried emotions and shed light on our sometimes inappropriate reactions to certain situations in present life.

Many problems in this life are connected with images and sensations from past lives. When you reexperience these memories fully, the problems in this life begin to disappear. For example, if you have problems in relationships, you will most likely see and experience scenes and images during a regression utilizing conscious breathing, that are connected to those same relationship problems. You are then able to let them go and transform them. You also will begin to perceive your problems in a different light, as you start to understand your present behavioral patterns, as they relate to past life circumstances.

During my first rebirthing experience, my intention was to try to reexperience the first two years of my life. For some reason, during several different previous hypnotic regressions, I had not been able to regress past age two. I hoped to reexperience my birth and perhaps part of my infancy. What occurred was totally unexpected. I regressed into a past life experience in Hiroshima, Japan, during the atom bomb blast in World War ll. The experience was very traumatic, and much emotion was released. As a result, I came to a greater understanding of the underlying reasons for my attitudes in this life and why I had manifested several specific diseases. I also understood that I had chosen that particular experience to learn certain lessons in that life. Reexperiencing my death, and the knowledge that I gained during that time period, enabled me to face the present with a great deal of confidence and hope for the future. My personal experiences with rebirthing have been very beneficial, because they have enabled me to release long and deeply buried emotions, while freeing up my psyche to new and more positive ways of being in the world. The additional insights into my motivations in and reactions to certain situations in life have also been of great benefit.

A storm of crying
clears the
pool of Regret
Nari

Rebirthing is a very powerful healing tool, and when used in combination with Reiki,many positive changes can occur. One example of this potent combination is as follows: During one of my trips abroad, I was approached by a young man with a severe stuttering problem. He asked me if I would treat him. My first inclination was to encourage him to take the Reiki class and learn to heal himself. My inner guidance, however, encouraged me to help him personally, so I made some time for an appointment. When he arrived for treatment, I started out with Reiki on his head. When I reached the throat chakra, he began to spasm and his arms and hands began to shake. Tremendous energy releases were surging through his body. My intuition lead me to direct him in a conscious breathing process. As he began the rhythmic breathing, the movements accelerated, and he began to have responses, similar to those that some people have in bioenergetic exercises. Later, after finishing this process, he even remembered a specific past life event which was directly connected with his stuttering. When the session was over, his stuttering was remarkably reduced. Although it was still there to some degree, he felt a great release and a lightening of his psyche. I encouraged him to use a set of creative visualizations and affirmations to fully release his old stuttering patterns. When I saw him a few days later, his speech was very much improved. Due to his willingness to heal himself, the combined tools of Reiki and Rebirthing helped a young man initiate some very powerful changes in his life. Anyone with the same willingness to allow growth and change in their life, will find Reiki and Rebirthing to be a very suitable combination.

There are many other therapies which may be used together with Reiki. I encourage you to use it in your area of expertise, and allow its supportive energies to assist you in the creation of your own healing form.

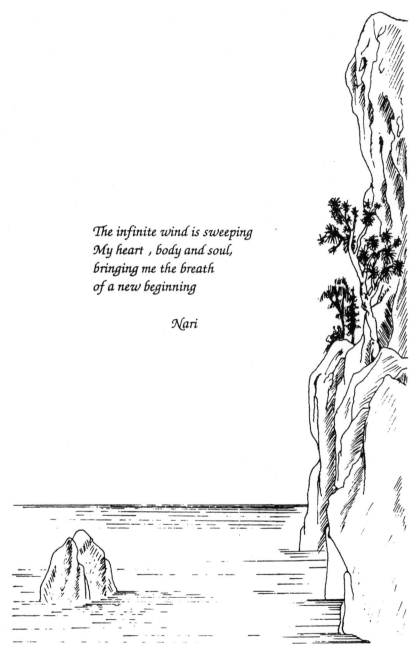

The infinite wind is sweeping
My heart , body and soul,
bringing me the breath
of a new beginning

Nari

108

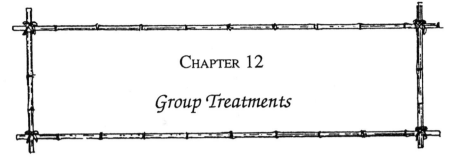

Group treatments are a wonderful way to share the Reiki energy among friends. I encourage my students to arrange get-togethers for this specific purpose. Group treatments are usually shorter than formal one-on-one treatments, as the full body is covered by several people. The experience of having ten to twelve hands on your body is quite enjoyable. The energy is also amplified as a result of so many channels tending to you at once.

During the First Degree Reiki class, I arrange six chairs around each massage table (or a comperable sized table covered with padding). One chair is placed at the head and one at the feet. The other chairs are arranged along the two sides of the table. One person starts out on the table and six more take different positions around the table. The person at the head of the table is the "leader" and watches the clock. Each time the person at the head changes hand position, each of the others also change position. I usually start with very short treatments. Each person has the opportunity to take a turn on the table and experience a ten minute treatment (five minutes on the front and five minutes on the back). Each person sitting (or standing, if more comfortable) around the table covers three positions on both sides of the body during the ten minute treatment. All changes in hand positions are coordinated with the person at the head of the table. A sort of "musical chairs" takes place each time the person on the table is completed. The person at the head then takes a turn on the table and the others all move to the next chair in a counterclockwise movement. Each person then has the opportunity to experience working on the different areas of the body, as well as, experiencing an assortment of different body types. As only 1 1/2 minutes is spent in each position, the students also begin to develop a sense that certain areas may not have received enough energy – that the body was still drawing energy when it was time to move on (the following day, when they give and receive a full hour treatment with a partner, they get the chance to feel the different levels of heat as they are perceived over the course of a full body treatment). The quick treatments enable a student to develop a kinesthetic sense of the body. Also, the feedback from the different recipients helps to verify for each Reiki healer that, yes their hands did indeed heat up in a certain area where large amounts of energy were being drawn.

Once the students have developed a kinesthetic sense of the body, I recommend longer group treatments, spending from three to five minutes in each position, or longer if desired or needed.

Group treatments are a very powerful tool for helping people with diseases such as cancer and AIDS. In Santa Fe, New Mexico, the Reiki Alliance established La Casa de Corazon (The House of the Heart), in 1987, for the treatment of AIDS patients. Two to three group and single treatments per day were administered to help stabilize the patients. Reiki practitioners around the world might consider establishing networks to perform treatments for AIDS and cancer patients. Hands on treatments in the hospitals would be most beneficial if permissible, and the other possibility of Second Degree level absentee healings could also be performed.

Second Degree group treatments can be used for more than just healing individuals. Group treatments can be sent to promote peace in war torn countries, to heal an area which has suffered from a natural disaster, to send healing energy to the ozone layer, and to offer loving vital energy to any situation which needs it. Again, as Reiki is drawn, not sent, only the energy needed will be drawn by each individual or situation. Reiki is an excellent tool to help heal the earth, which so desperately needs our attention now. As the planet provides us with an overflowing of abundance, taking the time to send it treatments is an excellent exchange of energy and a wonderful expression of gratitude. Whether group treatments are given to individuals, specific areas of the planet, or the entire planet as a whole, the healing which occurs as a result will directly affect us all. For each one of us to be whole, all must be made whole. The converse is true as well: For all of us to be whole, each individual must be made whole. Whereas the Eastern countries such as Japan have focused on the first premise with its concentration on the group, the West has focused on the second premise and the development of the individual. Both paths are correct in their own way. Reiki treatments can balance the two.

CHAPTER 13

Treating Infants, Plants, Animals, Food and Assorted Odds and Ends

Pregnant women enjoy Reiki treatments, because they help to alleviate some of the minor and major complaints of pregnancy, such as morning sickness in the first trimester, and later, lower back pain. Reiki also helps to soothe women as the emotions begin to fluctuate due to the large amount of hormones being released in the system. The infant itself appears to enjoys Reiki. During the time my sister was pregnant, the treatments seemed to energize her baby, as its feet would start to kick and little elbows would poke out. Also, the baby would tend to change positions more often during treatments, while there was still enough free space to move. We used Reiki on my sister during the entire birth process, and treated my niece directly after birth.

Reiki practitioners who are involved with gardening are well aware of the benefits that plants derive from being treated. Seeds that are treated before being planted, tend to grow into healthier plants than those which are not treated. Hold them between the palms of your hands and treat them as long as they draw energy. Seed sprouts in the earth can be treated by holding your hands just above them. Regular treatments given to your vegetable garden helps to produce an abundance of vital healthy plants. Flowers and shrubs do very well too when treated with Reiki. Blossoms tend to proliferate, and the growth of shrubs is accelerated. Cut flowers tend to last longer when supported with Reiki, and house plants also react with beneficial results.

Much has been written about the secret life of plants. Scientific tests have been done to show how plants react to our emotions, and to music. It has also been found that talking to plants helps to aid in the development of a healthy specimen. The great success of the Findhorn community in Northern Scotland is world renown. In a very baren wind swept coastal area, a group of people have successfully turned an otherwise undernourished land into a prolific garden paradise. By incorporating the help of nature spirits, they have successfully tuned in with their environment and have overcome otherwise insurmountable difficulties to produce a lavish abundance of plant growth. It seems that by the example of Findhorn, and other similar communities which have developed from its example, by communicating with the elementals of nature we can accomplish otherwise impossible tasks on the planet.

Second Degree practitioners might consider sending treatments to the elementals of certain plants in order to help them in their work on the Earth. The cooperation between humans and nature spirits may result in the rejuvenation of the entire ecological system.

Animals are appreciative recipients of Reiki energy, and most often become very calm and relaxed while treated. Occasionally you will find a rare animal who rejects the energy, and that must be respected. The average animal, however, will experience the same benefits that humans do. The fact that animals are healed with Reiki treatments tends to prove that the belief system has little effect on the outcome of the healing, although faith in any cure does help.

Animal anatomy is very similar to human anatomy, so, when treating a specific organ in an animal's body, you can judge its position fairly easily by its placement in your own body. Also, as with treating humans, special attention should be given to areas which draw larger amounts of energy. Covering the endocrine system, when possible, is also recommended.

If an animal is very restless, or it seems dangerous to treat with hands on, absentee healings can be utilized. Petting an animal before treatment is one way to soothe it. You can then follow your

114

intuition in the placement of your hands. Altogether, you will find Reiki a very practical tool for maintaining the health of your pets. Reiki can be used to energize an assortment of objects. Crystals have already been mentioned. Gem stones, and jewelry are also possibilities, along with an assortment of other objects. We must keep in mind that all matter is vibration at different levels of density – that everything on the physical plane is composed of universal life force energy in different phases of evolution. As all matter is vibration, Reiki can penetrate anything, much like the etheric substance of your body which permeates your environment. It is also possible to clear an environment such as a hotel room with Reiki energy, to remove any negative etheric substance.

On the more mundane level, cars and boats can also be treated. These objects actually tend to take on the etheric energy of their owners and become affected by our moods. Have you ever noticed that when you are in a negative or "down" cycle, your car tends to break down, or you blow out a sail? Boaters are especially aware of how their boats tend to take on an actual personality. Machines act as our mirrors as they become permeated with our energy over time. They become the anima to our animus or the animus to our anima. When the two are not in harmony, Reiki treatments are called for, because they can help you to avoid undesirable breakdowns and mechanical mishaps.

Finally, it should be mentioned that food can be enhanced by treating it with Reiki. In most countries around the world, people tend to eat an excessive amount of cooked or "dead" foods. In America alone, the average person eats 75% cooked food and only 25% raw food. In countries with the most centenarians, such as Russia, Bulgaria, the Hunzas in India, and some of the Mayan cultures, the people eat about a 73% raw food diet and 27% cooked food. The raw foods provide live enzymes which keep the body young and healthy and prevent the deterioration which causes quick aging in most of the human race. A raw food diet is an important factor in health. When you are in situations which prevent you from obtaining the correct amount of raw live foods, you can enhance your cooked food with the universal life force energy of Reiki. By just holding your hands above your plate you can treat your food, and afterwards, also treat your belly to aid in the process of digestion.

As we have seen in this chapter, all matter is composed of the Universal Life Force Energy at different levels of vibration. Reiki, which is a channeled and intensified form of this energy, can be used to energize not only living breathing life forms, but also "solid" matter. You are encouraged to allow your imagination free reign and to use your intuition to explore the endless possibilities.

CHAPTER 14

The Importance of an Energy Exchange

After his experience in the Beggars Quarter of Kyoto, Dr. Usui learned first hand about the importance of an exchange of energy for the healer's time. When he first became empowered to perform the miracle healings he had sought for so long, his initial thought was to move to the Beggars Quarter in true Christian style and serve the poor. His intention was to help heal them so that they could become responsible citizens, and enable them to hold a job to support themselves. What he discovered over time was that many returned after having experienced a taste of life on the outside, and decided that they didn't want the responsibility of caring for themselves. By just giving away healings, he had further impressed the beggar pattern in many of them. People needed to give back for what they received in order to fully appreciate what had been given.

As was discussed in Chapter Five, Usui thus discovered two very important factors: One, that a person should ask for a healing (It is not the job of any healer to try and help where healing is not wanted); and two, that there should be an exchange of energy for the healer's time (It is not right to keep someone feeling indebted for services rendered, thus the healee, by sharing energy in a variety of forms, frees himself of obligation).

The exchange of energy does not necessarily have to be in the form of money. It can be in the form of a trade of some sort. If the person requesting one or more treatments is a family member or very close friend, there is normally an exchange of energy taking place all of the time, so there need not be a request for specific reimbursement.

Not only should there be an exchange of energy for treatments, but there should also be an exchange of energy for Reiki classes. I seek students who are ready to receive the Reiki energy and are willing to earn it. It is important that a student appreciates and is prepared for the benefits of Reiki. The underlying principle is the same as that which Dr. Usui discovered after his years in the Beggars Quarter. He had seen many people come and go, and had also seen many return to their old ways. Usui decided to seek out people who really wanted to transform themselves. Christ's maxim, to "not throw pearls before swine," became clear. One should not waste precious time and energy sharing information or energy with those who are not interested or prepared to receive.

Another aspect of exchange of energy has to do with the concept of tithing. Much of the money that I earn in the West pays for my trips to underdeveloped countries. I feel that it is a good idea to tithe our abundance and share the Reiki energy with those less economically abundant than ourselves. Tithing must be done out of a deep sense of love, and not out of obligation, otherwise it will not have as profound of an effect. While I do it by teaching overseas, you, as an individual, can contribute by sharing your time and sending absentee treatments to different situations as mentioned in the discussion of group treatments in Chapter 12. To send treatments to helpless people, such as some-one in a coma, is one example. Although they cannot ask for a treatment, they will take only what they need, because Reiki is drawn, not sent. Also, by sending Reiki treatments to war and disaster ravaged areas of the Earth, we can help to create a more positive loving energy which will eventually engulf the entire planet.

Another important question which is often asked, is how does one become a professional Reiki practitioner? The answer is different in each country. In America, Physicians, Nurses, Massage Therapists, Physiotherapists, Chiropractors, Acupuncture Doctors, Naturopaths, Homeopaths, and Ayervedic Doctors all have license to touch the body and can readily blend Reiki with their treatments. Many psychologists are also adding Reiki to their practices, due to the powerful emotional healing technique introduced in Second Degree. For those others who find that they have a strong drive in this area, by obtaining a ministers license, you have the right to do spiritual healing and request donations. A specific fee cannot be charged, but you can suggest a donation. In West Germany, such a process is unfortunately not available. You must either obtain a Heil Praktiker's license, or you can use cards advertising Reiki as a Relaxation Technique, as long as you do not use the word therapy. It is your responsibility to find out the specific laws that affect the area in which you live.

As far as an exchange of energy is concerned, the fee for a Reiki treatment should be considered comparable to the fee for an hour of massage therapy in your area. One key piece of advice is to never make a diagnosis unless you are a doctor. If you strongly sense that something is very wrong, you may refer a person to a qualified doctor for a proper diagnosis. Also, never prescribe drugs or suggest that someone discontinue them. You can share other possibilities if you are so inclined.

Although one of the first premises of Reiki is that a person must ask for a treatment, you must not also feel obligated to oblige if you are not so inclined. It is very important to realize that sometimes people derive secondary benefits from illness. Although they may ask for a healing on a conscious level, or to put it bluntly, give "lip service" to wanting to be healed, they may not really want to be healed. For example, a spouse or child who frequently lacks attention from a mate or a parent, may find that all the attention that he or she receives while ill is a difficult thing to give up. If you treat someone for awhile, and your intuition begins to tell you that they are becoming overly dependent on you, and that they need to take full responsibility for their own healing, you should take steps to release them. One simple way to break this gently to a client is to tell them that your inner guidance has advised you that they are quite capable of healing themselves, and that there is nothing more that you can do for them at this time. You might suggest that they take a Reiki class and learn to treat themselves, or give them a creative visualization or affirmation that they can use. It is really important to know when it is time to release a client. For over and above giving treatments, we want to promote responsible, consciously aware individuals.

As we have seen, arranging an exchange of energy is an important part of the healing process. It saves people from the burden of obligation, and also it helps them to have an investment in the end result. The exchange should be in proportion to the person's income, and does not necessarily need to involve money. The give and take of Reiki, is truly one of its important assets. To live in a balanced, harmonious world, we must be comfortable with both giving and receiving. This is what exchange of energy is all about.

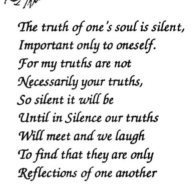

The truth of one's soul is silent,
Important only to oneself.
For my truths are not
Necessarily your truths,
So silent it will be
Until in Silence our truths
Will meet and we laugh
To find that they are only
Reflections of one another

Nari

CHAPTER 15

Treating Specific Disorders

When treating a variety of disorders, there are two basic guidelines to follow, as most pathologies fall under the two categories of acute and chronic disease. Acute problems, by definition, are of a short duration, and usually react in a different way to Reiki treatments than chronic problems which have a longer duration. The key difference between the two categories is that acute cases usually involve an immediate healing crisis, also called physical chemicalization, whereas chronic cases experience a healing crisis much later or not at all during the course of treatment.

When a client with a chronic disease, such as arthritis, begins a series of Reiki treatments, the pain usually dissipates rapidly during the first few sessions. If the treatments are given over a period of several weeks, the pain and swelling generally continue to disappear until the disease reaches the point of physical chemicalization. It is at this stage that the client may experience a relapse, and feel the effects of the disease even more painfully than before the beginning of treatment. This is a sign that you have reached the final level of toxic build-up, where the last vestiges of the dis-ease are entrenched. As the Reiki energy makes contact with this final layer of toxins, the reaction resembles the lighting of a match. The sudden intense flame, which occurs immediately, burns away the match head. Likewise, the powerful energy of Reiki, when exposed to the disease, purges it with a strong current of life force energy.

Physical chemicalization is an unpleasant but favorable symptom. It is important at this point to explain the process to your client, and to increase the number of treatments until the healing crisis has passed. It should be noted that occasionally a healing crisis does not occur and the symptom may just dwindle as the layers of toxins slowly pass away. Therefore, in chronic cases it is appropriate not to mention beforehand the possibility of physical chemicalization, as it may never arise in a noticeable manner. Thus it is better to wait, and if it does occur you can assure the patient that it is a positive sign. Otherwise, avoid projecting unnecessary symptoms onto your client.

Acute cases are an entirely different matter. Usually, the person is in pain, as the disease is relatively new. Hopefully, the patient has already visited a doctor, and your function is only to accelerate the healing process. If not, and the problem is serious, it is generally a good idea to refer them to a qualified physician. When treating an acute problem, Reiki treatments often tend to initially intensify the pain, because a large amount of healing energy drawn to the problem area creates a sense of pressure. This symptom usually dissipates within two to three days, and relief of the problem is usually very rapid. Acute symptoms react this way to many different methods of healing.

A few years ago, while I was volunteering in the clinic of a Mexican Spiritualist healer, a young woman was brought in a few days after childbirth. As she and her husband were very poor, and couldn't afford a hospital or midwife, the child had been born at home. Later, she developed an infection, most likely from left over fetus material. She was again rejected by the local hospitals, and was carried into the clinic by her husband in a great deal of pain. After she was treated, the healer mentioned that she might feel a bit more pain for the next couple of days, but would soon begin to feel better on or about the third day. What I discovered later, is that there seems to be a lag time of approximately three days for healings on the etheric body to finally affect the physical body. Most spiritual and psychic healing methods work in this way. With Reiki there is no specific "lag time" as it is focused into both the physical and etheric bodies during treatment. As the healee draws the energy in, he/she also determines the length of treatment needed.

Whenever you are dealing with an acute healing problem, it is wise to inform the person that they might experience more discomfort for the first couple of days, until the symptoms begin to dissipate. Unlike dealing with chronic problems, which may or may not manifest a healing crisis, acute cases seem to produce more intense symptoms during the initial healing phase. Thus, it is wise to have the person prepared by properly informing them of the common reactions to such cases.

Occasionally, you may receive a complaint of pain or discomfort from a person who has been treated and wasn't suffering from any ailment beforehand. People sometimes have diseases or illnesses building up in their bodies, and are totally unaware of it. Reiki treatments can accelerate the healing energy in that area, which in turn, may be experienced as pain or discomfort. A primary example occured after I had just received First Degree Reiki. A very close friend was visiting from overseas, and I had given her a Reiki treatment early in the morning. After I went to work that evening, I received a call from the emergency room at the local hospital. My friend had begun to experience intense pain and she had asked a friend of mine to take her to the hospital. Initially, she was misdiagnosed as having a uterine infection, but later it was discovered that she had kidney stones. Apparently the Reiki treatment accelerated the healing process by moving the stones through the kidneys. It gave my friend her first awareness that a problem even existed. It is also important to keep in mind that in a case like this, Reiki is drawn, not sent. Although I felt sorry about my friend's pain, her body did draw energy in the appropriate amount that she needed. The whole incident later helped her to reconsider her diet and make healthy changes in her life. From this incident and other similar ones, it can be seen that Reiki does indeed accelerate the healing process of the body. Another illustration that I like to give my students is the example of an infected cut on the skin. As the white blood cells rush to the infection and devour all of the invading bacteria, the feeling of pressure from all of the healing activity translates into pain.

Therefore, unpleasant physical symptoms often are only signs that the body is operating properly in accomplishing all of the tasks needed to complete the healing process.

When treating different disorders, it is important to remember that Reiki can penetrate any solid matter, such as cloth, wood, or steel. Reiki can also penetrate a plaster cast, while treating a broken bone. It is wise to wait until after a bone is properly set to treat it directly. If you need to treat a person who feels uncomfortable with having someone touch them physically, you can transmit Reiki by allowing your hands to hover just above the body. Reiki treatments are highly recommended for patients who are going to have surgery. It is best to treat them only before and after the operation, because Reiki can accelerate the effect of the anesthesia on the body and cause it to wear off prematurely.

Mrs. Takata taught a simple pattern of hand positions which follow the endocrine system. She often added a few of her own positions as I and others have done. You can use them for self-treatments or for working on others: Begin by placing your palms over the eyes. This position should also cover the sinuses. The second position covers the temples, next the ears, and the fourth, the occipital lobes at the base of the skull. For the fifth position, place one hand over both occipital lobes and the other over the forehead. This position covers both the pineal and pituitary glands, and the hypothalamus. It is a good position for relieving headaches, stress, and tension. The next position is the throat, which can be covered by placing each hand at either side of the neck, or as I prefer, with one hand behind the upper neck and one gently placed over the top front of the throat (covering many of the lymph glands below the jaw on either side of the wind pipe). The seventh position covers the thyroid and thymus glands, followed by the heart and solar plexus (adrenal glands). At this point I like to add to Mrs. Takata's technique and include the liver-just below the lower right ribcage, the upper lungs (one hand on each lung), and the spleen-pancreas area opposite the liver. I now return to the basic pattern with the hara or Chi point – three finger widths below the navel. Next cover the ovaries for women (just above the pubic bone), or just above the lymph nodes at the top of each thigh for men. The knees are then treated, as they hold our fear of change, and fear of death of the ego. Finally, you can complete the front with the feet. On the back, work from the shoulders down to the sacrum and finish with the spinal balance.

Other areas of the body can be included as well. It is best to use your intuition to guide you as to what is appropriate. Whenever there is a specific disorder, such as diabetes, you should treat the appropriate internal organs that are affected by the disease, which, in this case, would be the pancreas. If there is a heart problem, of course you would focus on the heart. Also, it is good to spend at least thirty minutes per day on the specific disease areas of the body, such as a malignant tumor in the case of cancer. Try to spend time on the endocrine system and place special emphasis on the thymus gland, which we know has a powerful effect on the immune system. Again, you should use your intuition to guide you, and leave your hands on areas which continue to draw energy, for as long as possible. Signals which tell you when it is time to change position are varied. You might see or feel the patient take a deep sigh of relief, feel the heat begin to decrease in your hands, or feel the pulsations or tingling subside. Actually, just an intuitive sense that it's time to change positions is quite adequate. The average time to spend in each area is approximately three to five minutes, but can be extended as needed.

Finally, when treating any person, no matter how emotionally bonded you may be, you must not have any attachments to the results of your healing.

One of the most difficult lessons that I have learned as a healer has been to let go and allow each person to decide whether they want to get well or stay sick, to live or to die.

A few years ago, when my mother contracted cancer, the first treatments that I sent seemed to help heal the initial surgery very quickly. Soon after, to my great disappointment, she chose to try chemotherapy along with a Macrobiotic diet and Gerson therapy.

I continued to send treatments from California to Germany. As I am an empath and can feel many people's symptoms in my own body, I could tell every time she was on chemotherapy. I had tried to dissuade her gently as I had watched other friends become cured from cancer by chemotherapy and then die from the side effects of the treatments. When I could see that she was firm in her decision, I supported her totally, because I felt that she needed all of the positive energy that she could get. A couple months later, when planning my trip to visit several of the Brazilian psychic surgeons, I called her and encouraged her to come along. Again she declined as she was going to try some other new chemotherapy in Southern Germany. As it turned out, she died while I was in Brazil. She made contact with me there, and with the help of Second Degree Reiki, I was able to help her through the dying process from six thousand miles away. I will never forget that period of time. It was one of the most spiritual experiences of my life. Mixed with the sadness and grief of losing my mother in the physical form, came the realization, through very powerful verifications, that she never really died. She simply passed on to another form. I had wanted her to come and join us in our adventure in Brazil, and that is indeed what transpired. She remained in her astral body for a few weeks until the whole family could meet in the United States and release their grief, and then wish her well on her way.

The feeling of treating someone with Reiki during the process of dying is a very spiritual experience. I felt so privileged to be able to be with my mother during such an important transition. The only other experience that could compare was participating in the birth of my sister's first child, for birth and death are both transitions. The love energy inherent in each experience is so overwhelming that words cannot begin to express the true feeling. The essential factor in each is that you are dealing with the whole perfect person in the true sense of the word. Babies are born as perfect whole beings, and during the death process all of the old dross is shed, revealing the true beauty of the person in transition.

In actual fact, each person that we treat is a perfect whole being, and the "disorder" that we see is just an illusion waiting to be pealed away at the right time, when the lesson of the dis-ease is completed. We as healers are simply here to support and encourage others in this awesome process. It is indeed a great privilege to be a healer, as we get to glimpse behind the mask at the true perfection of each person. Our job is to help them see that same perfection. Reiki is a wonderful tool to help us reach that goal.

Death is but an awakening from
The dreams of the night.
A returning of the soul to the light

Nari

CHAPTER 16

Body Psychology - How and Where Emotions are stored in the Body

Most people, when considering the study of psychology relate to the brain as being the center of mental activity. Indeed, the brain is the physical organ which registers and retains thoughts and memories, much like a computer. However, the mind itself actually functions through the etheric (bioplasmic) body and leaves its impressions throughout the entire physical structure. You may have heard the maxim: "You are what you eat". This might also be stated, "You are what you think." In other words, the matter that we take into our bodies helps to shape our physical structures, and by the same token, the thoughts we project, and the emotional reactions that pass through our bodies, also affects its form and texture. Thus the body is a reflection of the mind, and in turn, as the body develops in certain ways, the mind will act as a reflection of the body. The body's tissues will actually adjust their size and texture according to the quality of emotions and thoughts passing through it. Positive energy will help to keep the body flexible and supple, whereas suppressed actions of desires will tend to create energy blocks in the etheric and then physical bodies. Blocked energy will actually form rigidity in the tissue. The rigidity then collects and helps to form "Body Armor", a term used by Wilhelm Reich to illustrate the excess tissue which builds up to create a psychological "protective" barrier. Massage therapists experience this daily in their clients as tightness in the trapezius muscles, where we have literally taken the weight of the world on our shoulders, and in assorted other areas, according to our particular body psychology.

131

Nose
- related to heart
  (coloration and bulbousness)
- sense and smell, sexual response
- self recognition

Mouth
- survival issues
- how we take in nourishment
  security
- capacity to take in new ideas

Forehead
- intellectual expression

Neck
- thought and emotions come
  together
- stiffness is due to withheld
  statements

Arms and hands
- are extensions of the heart center
- express love and emotion

Solar Plexus (diaphragm)
- power issues
- emotional control issues
  power wisdom center

Genitals
- related to root chakra containing
  Kundalini
- survival issues
- fear of life

Knees
- fear of death
- fear of death of the old-self or ego
- fear of change

Face
- expresses the various "masks" of our
  personality
- shows how we "face" the world

Eyes
- show how we see the world
- nearsighted is more withdrawn
- farsighted is less inner oriented
- windows of the soul

Brow
- intuitive center
- emotional expression

Ears
- our capacity to hear
- have acupuncture points for every
  area of the body

Jaw
- tension indicates blockage of emotional
  and verbal communication
- fear or ease of expression

Chest
- relationship issues
- heart and love emotions
- respiration and circulation

Abdomen
- seat of the emotions
- contains our deepest feelings
- center of sexuality
- digestive system

Thigh
- personal strength
- trust in one's own abilities
- fear of inadequate strength

Feet
- show if we are grounded
- connected with reaching our goals
- fear of completion

132

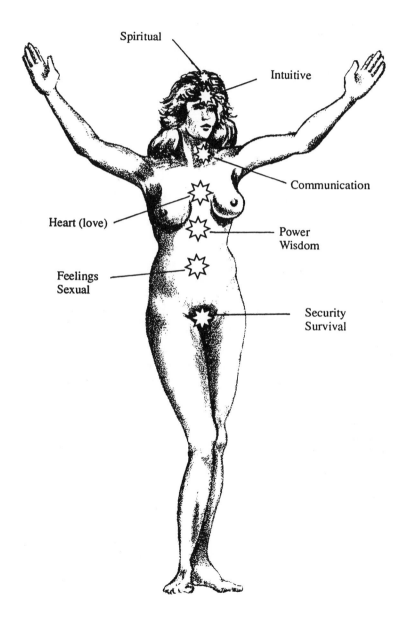

Spiritual

Intuitive

Communication

Heart (love)

Power
Wisdom

Feelings
Sexual

Security
Survival

Hands
- giving and receiving
- holding on to reality
- reaching goals
- fear of action

Forearm
- means of attaining goals
- fear of inferiority

Arms
- express the heart center, love
- enable us to move and
- connect in the external world

Upper arm
- strength to act
- fear of being discouraged

Elbow
- connects the strength of
  the upper arms to the
  action of the forearm

Upper back
- (particularly between
  the shoulder blades) we
  carry stored anger

Lower back
- junction between lower and
  upper body movement
- men store a lot here due to
  the storing of emotions in
  the belly

Gluteus muscles
- Holding in emotions – not
  releasing and letting go
- anal blockage

Abductors
- inner thigh)
- contain sexually charged issues

Ankles
- create balance

Shoulders
- where we carry the weight of
  the world
- fear of responsibility
- women store a lot here

Back
- where we store all of our unconscious
  emotions, and excess tension

Pelvis
- seat of Kundalini energy
- root of basic survival needs
  and actions

Hamstrings
- self control issues
- letting go

Lower leg
- enables movement toward goals
- fear of action

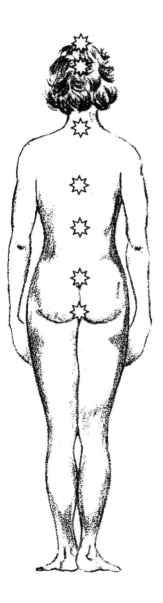

FRONT/BACK DIVISION

Front: our mirror to the world
— your social mask
— contains the emotional
  issues of daily life, such as:
  Love, desire, sadness, joy,
  concern, etc.
— heart "pain" is stored in the
  chest, between the ribs and
  the insides of the shoulders.
  Much emotion is also stored
  in the belly

Back: stores many of our unconscious thoughts and emotions
— where we hide issues we are
  not prepared to handle
— our emotional disposal area
  for all the things we don't
  want to acknowledge
— a lot of fear and anger is
  stored between the shoulder
  blades, and along the
  spinalis muscle on either
  side of the spine

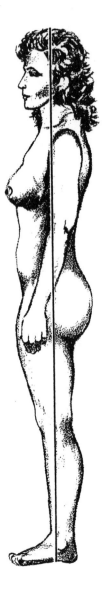

RIGHT-LEFT DIVISION

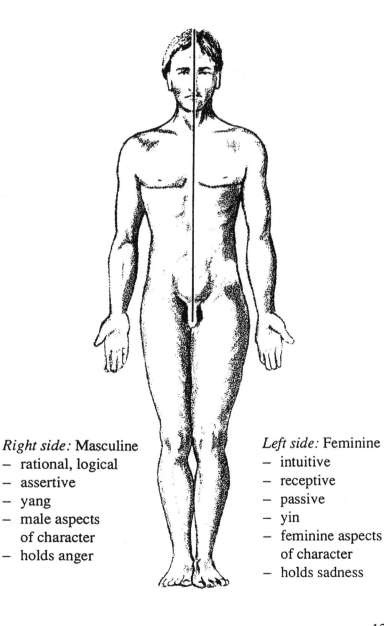

Right side: Masculine
- rational, logical
- assertive
- yang
- male aspects
  of character
- holds anger

Left side: Feminine
- intuitive
- receptive
- passive
- yin
- feminine aspects
  of character
- holds sadness

$$\frac{HEAD}{BODY} \quad DIVISION$$

$$\frac{Human}{Animal}$$

$$\frac{Mind}{Body}$$

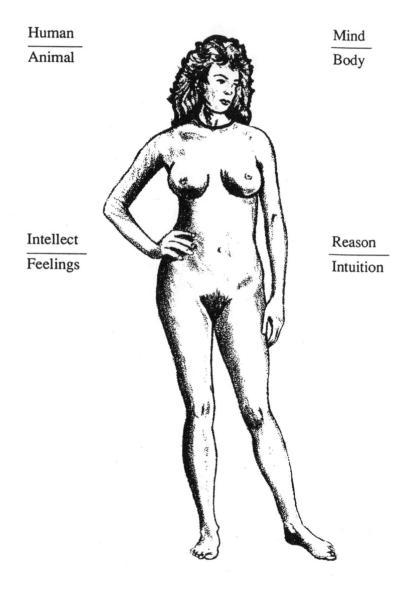

$$\frac{Intellect}{Feelings}$$

$$\frac{Reason}{Intuition}$$

$$\frac{TOP}{BOTTOM} \quad DIVISION$$

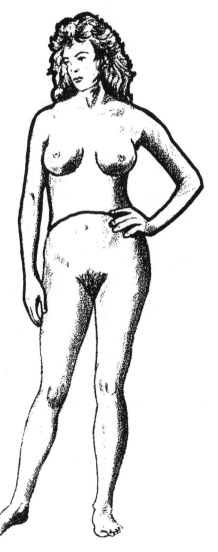

Small Top
Large Bottom
(found most often in females)
— finds difficulty in
   socializing, outward
   expression, interpersonal
   communications,
   self-assertion, and taking
   action
— tendency toward privacy,
   stable, homey and well
   grounded
— passive personality

Large Top
Small Bottom
Found most often in males)
— overdeveloped in ability to
   be assertive, social
   expressive, extroverted
— lack of strength and courage
   with respect to emotional
   stability and support
— active personality

LIMB/TORSO DIVISION

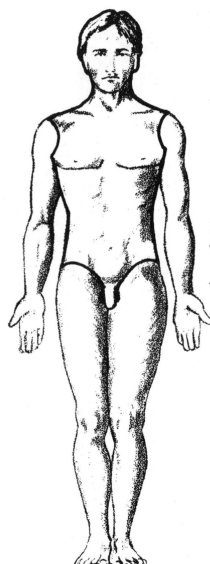

Limbs
– are the vehicles for making
  contact with the outside
  world – they allow us to
  move in space
– most active parts of the
  body in regard to the outside
  world

Torso
– is the "core of the body, the
  center of the private self
– very inactive regarding the
  outside world – tends to be
  more reflective, focused on
  the self

Each body part has a unique story to tell, according to its special bodymind function. The first two charts help illustrate the different types of emotions which are held in specific areas of the body. Note that there is also a definite connection between the chakras or seven main energy centers, and the types of emotions that are stored in the corresponding areas of the body. Just as the endocrine system corresponds directly to the charkras, or energy centers, the Mental and Emotional Bodies are also closely linked.

As can be seen in the previous two charts, the body is a true expression of the mind and emotions. In addition to factors such as heredity, environment, nutrition, and daily physical activity, the powerful emotions and thought forms which move through the body help to mold its very fabric and posture.

In different countries, due to the growing interest of peoples around the world to understand essential body-mind functions, I have taught a weekend workshop combining basic body psychology, and an introduction to emotional release work to help people discover certain tools for cleansing blocked areas of the body. Initially I discuss the ideal physical structure as promulgated by Ida Rolf, the developer of Rolfing. According to Rolf, a person with a healthy Body/Mind structure, when standing erect, will show upon examination that his or her ears are directly above the shoulders, the shoulders are centered *over* the hips, the hips are directly over the knees and the knees over the ankles. If any of these areas are out of alignment, we can readily begin to note certain inferences about the person's personality or character type.

Dr. Rolf, a biochemist and physiologist who had studied muscle tissue and its various formations on the human body, noticed that emotional as well as physical traumas had a direct effect on the tightening and rigidification of the muscular and myofascial tissues of the body. She observed that fear, grief and anger, as they passed through the body, would cause the muscles to flex in certain "protective" postures. If the person repeated these postures several times, they would begin to rigidify, and the person would then start to assume the pysical attitude to the particular emotion. When this occurred, the natural alignment of the body was disrupted, and an overall inflexibility and gravitational imbalance would set in. Thus a habit pattern was formed and the muscular arrangement became permanent.

There are certain common divisions in physical structure which seem to occur often, and which help simplify the understanding of body psychology. The previous five illustrations were inspired by the book *Bodymind* by Ken Dychtwald, which is listed in the recommended reading as a source of in depth information on this subject.

To correct misalignments in structure, Dr. Rolf developed a 10-hour (ten session) process involving deep manipulation of the myo-facial layers in order to realign the body to a properly balanced whole. Over the years, as she refined her technique, she began to notice that people experienced a lot of emotional releases during the course of her work. In addition, it was clear that many different people all seemed to hold the same types of emotions in the same areas of the body. It also became clear that not only did negative emotion help to create rigid body armor in the course of daily life, but in the process of her work, she also began to see that a rigid posture (or body armor) created by previous emotional states, would also perpetuate these same emotions. Thus the mind and emotions affected the body, and in turn, the body structure could affect the mind and resulting emotions. As she released the rigid body armor and inappropriate postures through her work, the emotions stored in the structure of the body were also released, allowing the individual a new lightness of being, no longer burdened by the waste products of previous negative experience.

Rolf's work inspired not only physiotherapists and massage therapists, but in addition psychologists were drawn to her work by the obvious implications of possible and profound psychological changes inherent in her work. Many offshoots of her work appeared in the 1970s including Psycho-Structural Balancing, Aston Patterning, and Hellerwork.

While all of the variations of Rolf's work were developing, other healers were beginning to see the extreme usefulness of Acupressure points in the area of emotional release work. Chris Griscom of Galisteo, New Mexico, who has become well known for her work in past life regression, is one of a group of people who rediscovered the usefulness of the acupuncture meridians in the release of stored emotional blocks. Actually this knowledge has existed for thousands of years and has been used in several of the Eastern cultures. While the Chinese mapped out the energy meridians of acupuncture and explored the movement of the "chi", in India the yogis explored the etheric body which is energized by „prana" and carried through channels called „nadis". Several different forms of Yoga are aimed at "burning up" the energy blocks which prevent the flow of prana through the nadis. Chua Ka, an ancient and very deep form of Mongolian self-massage, helped warriors release their fears before going into battle by removing long held emotional blocks.

Most of the different forms of emotional release work focus on increasing the amount of life force energy in order to push up against any blocked channels in the subtle bodies. As the life force energy comes up against a block, the resistance which occurs sets off a high pitched vibratory state in the body. All the bodily systems are in turn affected which helps to stimulate and re-create the original trauma which created the blockage. The person then re-experiences the feelings associated with that event in the form of verbal discharge and possibly even an orgastic response (a physical reaction described by Bioenergetics). Rebirthing, which was discussed in Chapter 11, also employs an increase in vital energy through the vehicle of conscious breathing, in order to create the vibratory pressure needed to break through blocks.

The different schools of emotional release work all share a common goal, which is to initiate a cathartic release of emotional energy at a level beyond the functoning of the intellectual and rational faculties. Such a release helps to purge long accumulated trauma, and is equivalent to Janov's "primal scream". Technique is not necessarily an essential factor in reaching this goal, as the result is more often due to the readiness of the recipient's psyche to release such energy. A less than cathartic release where the person is still in conscious control yet is verbalizing emotion, perhaps experiencing body twitching or involuntary movements, is also helpful, as this may be the extent to which a person is prepared to release.

Some important factors which promote a successful emotional release sesson are as follows:

The practitioner should have a solid background in his or her technique, along with a deep understanding of the essentials of body psychology. Ideally the practitioner should acquire plenty of experience in not only helping others through release work, but also in completing a significant number of emotional clearings on oneself. In other words, in order to relate properly and create the feeling of a safe environment for cathartic release, there needs to be an empathetic sense of trust and security between both the healee and the practitioner. Empathy is a result of having shared similar personal experiences – an essential ingredient for a successful session.

There are a variety of techniques which help to promote a pressurized, high vibratory rate for intense emotional release. Such tools as conscious breathing, pressure points on certain parts of the body, visualizaton, and exercises such as those in Bioenergetics all help to move energy.

As I mentioned in Chapter 11, I often use Reiki in conjunction with Rebirthing. Another powerful tool to add to these two are pressure points on the body, which are located in commonly blocked areas.

At the beginning of Past Life Seminars where I utilize conscious breathing as the main tool for regresson, I generally give a brief overview of body psychology and encourage the participants to evaluate each other. Bodies are examined to determine where each individual is holding the most energy and just what pressure point might help to release the blockage. You may want to do the same. Take the time to evaluate your body with the help of a friend. Try to examine which areas have the most blockage and determine which emotional release points would have the greatest effect on your particular body type. You can refer to diagrams 15 and 16 as a guide. I suggest that you acquire the help of a professional rebirther/bodyworker and discuss your particular holding areas, and the present issue you would like to examine which is most affecting your life. With the use of conscious breathing you can then help guide your rebirther into specific pressure points in your body. After you have become familiar with the rebirthing process, you can begin to rebirth yourself. You can utilize the following technique on yourself as stated, or help guide an assistant during your own process:

It is wise to use most of the pressure points shown in the diagrams by starting at the feet and moving slowly up the body. Always exert pressure gently as the healee inhales, and maintain pressure or loosen if necessary on the exhale. As you come to important blockage points, you might try to exert a bit more pressure, yet at the same time, be sure that pressure doesn't build up to the point that it cant't get through the narrowed channel. Keep the energy flowing around the block and move back and forth on the body as necessary. Allow the energy to move – don't force it. When certain areas are not flowing, focus on the main pressure points in that area, such as the pelvis and thigh for the leg, or the shoulder for the arm.

Avoid too much talking unless appropriate. Engaging the intellect tends to detract from the process. Wait until the emotions have been released before asking too many questions. As the energy moves through the body you may note certain symptoms such as twitching, spasms etc. The healee may even cry when energy is released in the throat chakra. Allow the energy to take it's natural course. If an intense cathartic reaction occurs and you are acting as the guide, be sure to stay very grounded and focus on protecting the person from bodily harm or prolonged withholding of the breath. There is little or no facilitating needed at this point. Your

EMOTIONAL RELEASE POINTS

Third Eye
T.M.J.

Scaleness

Main shoulder point

Rib attachment to sternum

Solar Plexus

Press into rib cage

Inside Pelvic Bone

Bladder Alarm Point

Attachment of adductors

Halfway up thigh

Located at adductor attachment

Stomach 36

Liver source point

Start on vortex points

Begin at feet and
work up the body

146

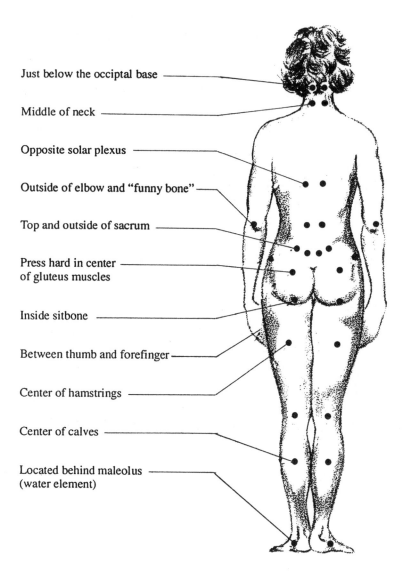

Just below the occiptal base

Middle of neck

Opposite solar plexus

Outside of elbow and "funny bone"

Top and outside of sacrum

Press hard in center
of gluteus muscles

Inside sitbone

Between thumb and forefinger

Center of hamstrings

Center of calves

Located behind maleolus
(water element)

intuition will tell you when the process has ended, or the healee will begin to engage in conscious interaction. If necessary, you can end the process by asking questions such as: What are you experiencing?, What are you seeing?, How are you doing?, in order to activate the intellect. After the emotional release is complete, you may want to share your experience with your rebirther, or if you are acting as the facilitator, you should allow the person to process his or her experience.

Emotional release work is a powerful tool for cleansing the energy body, however it does not help to reprogram ingrained habits which are associated with the release. To reeducate old subconscious patterns, I recommend using a 40-day program of affirmations which deal directly with the issue or issues which have been released. It takes at least 40 days to reprogram the subconscious, thus a 15 minute per day meditation utilizing appropriate affirmations in recommended.

We have reached the point in time where we must become clear and whole as a group in order to assist in the healing of the planet. As individuals we can take the first step by initiating our own cleansing processes through the clearing of the emotional body. In time, the resulting amplification of our vibratory frequencies will return us to our original state as true beings of light – whole and complete in harmony with the Universal Life Force.

CHAPTER 17

Reiki's Place in the Evolution of Consciousness

In today's open climate, in which people are searching for alternative solutions to many of life's problems, there is an increased awareness that healing takes place on more than a physical level. The power of mind integrated with matter is becoming more self-evident as thousands of people continue to share in the experience of firewalking, and powerful spiritual healing. These circumstances are providing people with an opportunity to wake up – to become more consciously aware, and to begin to break out of the mold of race mind consciousness. The old denial patterns and fears, which have been passed down for centuries from generation to generation, are slowly disappearing as we begin to sense the new vibratory frequency of love on the planet and adjust ourselves accordingly to it. We can no longer separate ourselves from each other and survive. We have created a situation where we must choose to cooperate or die. The old unconscious pattern of separation is fading away as we move toward a new collective consciousness of peace and harmony.

It is my feeling that all dis-ease is caused by negative emotions, due to a basic guilt of separation from God (All Mind) – by a false ego, unhappy or impatient, that feels "life isn't going my way". If one can for a moment escape the self-centered ego which is always tooting its own horn, one may become aware that we are not separated from God or the All Mind (our true-self and the true-selves of others); that indeed we truly are at one with the Universe (not separate). Through such a recognition, all blessings (healings) flow. Healing occurs through remembrance. Indeed, remembering who we truly are is the key to self-healing. Remebering where our emotions first got out of hand and reacted on the physical body is another important clue to discovering our specific misunderstandings which also relate back to the initial feeling of separateness. A quantum leap in the consciousness of mankind is now needed to defeat this old feeling of separation.

Reiki is a powerful tool which can help the individual release this sense of separaton. As the 21-day cleanse process commences after the First Degree Class, many old emotional blocks begin to be released. Intuition also becomes heightened, helping the individual to become more finely tuned to the higher self.

By amplifying the vibratory rate of the body, Reiki enables each person to channel larger amounts of energy, and also raises the vibratory level of the planet as a whole.

As Reiki is a tool of empowerment, it provides each individual with an opportunity to strip away the veils over consciousness which tend to hinder a clear perception of Truth. As we seek through inner work to develop greater conscious awareness, and a deeper level of communication with the Higher Self, we will see the resulting effect of these veils being lifted away and the state of Emanence made manifest.

Word List

ACUTE: Severe but of short duration (referring to disease).

ATTUNEMENTS: Special Reiki initiations which raise the vibratory rate of the body, and open a specific healing channel in the chakras.

ASTRAL BODY: One of the subtle bodies just one frequency higher than the etheric body, also closely linked to the emotions.

AURA: A subtle, invisible essence that emanates from humans, animals and other bodies

BIOENERGETIC EXERCISES: These were developed by Alexander Lowen, one of Wilhelm Reich's students. They are designed to generate electromagnetic energy in the body in order to move and release blockage.

BIOPLASMIC BODY: The Russian term for the etheric body or L-field.

CAUSAL FACTOR: Relates to the cause of disease – also the divine law of cause and effect. The causal body itself is one of the subtle bodies which stores all of our experiences from many different lifetimes.

CENTER: To place one's consciousness in the hara or belly chakra, to release the intellect and be at one with the All-Mind.

CHAKRAS: Are the energy centers located in the etheric body. They are closely linked to the endocrine system of the physical body.

CHANNEL (verb): To act as a human vehicle for the receiving and sending of information from any aspect of the All-Mind (your own higher self, spirit guide, etc.).

CHANNEL (noun): A person who has emptied oneself to allow an alternate form of consciousness to flow through.

CHRONIC: Lasting a long time (in reference to disease).

CRYSTAL GRIDWORK: A geometric pattern or layout of crystals which is used to enhance or amplify healing and meditation.

DIS-EASE: An alteration of the living body that impairs its functioning due to it being "Ill at ease". Such a state creates a health challenge for personal growth and new learning.

ELEMENTALS: Are repetitive thought forms which have taken on a life force of their own. Elementals can be seen by psychics in many different shapes and sizes (different than nature spirits).

ENERGY BLOCK: Refers to a point in both the etheric and physical bodies where energy has accumulated and cannot flow, due to disharmony in the body.

ETHERIC BODY: The bioplasmic body or energetic counterpart of the physical body, also known as the L-field.

EXORCISM: A ritual performed on behalf of people who are thought to be possessed by evil spirits, in an effort to drive the spirits out.

HEALING: A major or minor change which helps restore health.

KIRLIAN PHOTOGRAPHY: A special process developed by Semyon Kirlian in Russia, to record on film the corona discharge, or aura, of the subject.

L-FIELD: The "field of life" discovered by Burr and Northrup, also the etheric or bioplasmic body.

PATTERNS (old behavior): Recurring behavior caused by habit, and often initiated by certain reactions to situations in the individual's past history.

PHYSICAL CHEMICALIZATION: The final release of toxins which cause disease. It is often associated with a healing crisis in both acute and chronic cases.

PLASMATIC STREAMING: A release of energy through the system when an energy block is unclogged – also known as a "Kundalini rush".

PROCESS (to) - (verb): To digest or integrate information or therapy.

PSYCHIC HEALING: Healing which is performed through the projection of vibrations or energy, often at a distance.

PSYCHIC SURGERY: A form of psychic healing which focuses on the adjustment of the etheric body for healing purposes, and often has an outward appearance similar to actual surgery.

SUBTLE BODY: Any of the invisible (to normal eyesight) energy bodies (etheric, causal, and astral) of a higher vibratory frequency than the physical body.

VIBRATORY LEVEL: Refers to the various frequencies at which energy oscillates.

About the Author

Paula C Horan Ph.D.
P.O. Box 159
Rockport, WA 98283

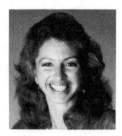

Paula Horan Ph . D. is a psychologist, lecturer, author, and human potential seminar leader. An inspirational teacher, she spends most of her time on the international circuit training people in a broad range of subjects.

Paula Horan exemplifies the traits of the new 21st century renaissance woman. Having previously completed a variety of careers as drama teacher, counsellor, professional dancer, systems management coordinator, and spa director and lecturer aboard ship, she perceived a body of knowledge developing, which helped provide keys to the unlocking of the inner-self. From this storehouse of knowledge and experience, Paula created a series of workshops and seminars that are well received by people from a variety of backgrounds.

Paula offers a wealth of knowledge in the area of self-healing, as she at one time cured herself of both a breast tumor and grand mal epileptic seizures. In 1986 she completed her study of a Mexican Spiritualist psychic surgeon, and conducted a survey tour of Spiritist healers in Brazil. Her exploration of vibrational medicine led her to Reiki, a very powerful tool for personal healing and transformation. Since that time she has committed her life to training people in Reiki to help them raise the vibratory level of the body, and promote greater conscious awareness, and The Core Empowerment Training, about which she co-authored a book by the some title. Paula appreciates comments from her readers. Any inquiries regarding Reiki, The Core Empowerment Training, or Firewalk seminars may be sent to the above address.

Recommended Reading

CHAPTER 1

Arnold, L. and Nevius, S. *The Reiki Handbook A Manual for Students and Therapists of the Usui Shiki Ryoho System of Healing.* Harrisburg, PA: Psi Press, 1982.

Baginski, B. and S. Sharamon *Reiki – Universal Life Energy.* Mendocino, CA: Life Rhythm Publishing, 1988.

Moss, T. *The Body Electric.* Los Angeles: J.P. Tarcher, Inc., 1979.

Ray, B. *The Reiki Factor.* Smithtown, NY: Expositions Press, 1982.

For Life Energy Interpretation Using Kirlian Photography for Healing contact: Dr. Bara H. Fischer, P.O. Box 8160, Santa Fe, NM 87504 (505) 984-9788

CHAPTER 4

Meek, G. *Healers and the Healing Process.* Wheaton, Illinois: Quest Books, 1977.

Tiller, W. "The Positive and Negative Space/Time Frames as Conjugate Systems" Fulture Science. Edited by Krippner and White. Garden City, NJ: Doubleday and Co., 1977.

CHAPTER 5

Price, R. *The Abundance Book,* Austin, Texas: Quartus Books, 1987.

Price, R. *The Manifestation Process: 10 Steps to the Fulfillment of Your Desires* Austin, Texas: Quartus Books 1983

Price, R. *The Superbeings* Austin, Texas: Quartus Books, 1986.

CHAPTER 10: Removing Energy Blocks

Horan, Paula *A Phenomenological Case Study of A Mexican Spiritualist. Psychic Surgeon.* (Dissertation) San Diego, CA: The University for Humanistic Studies, 1986.

Uhl, M. *Chakra Energy Massage.* Lotus Light Publications, P.O. Box 2, Wilmot, WI 53192.

Using Color and Sound

David, W. *The Harmonics of Sound, Color and Vibration: A System for Self-Awareness and Soul Evolution.* Marina Del Ray, CA: DeVorss & Co. 1980.

Dinshah, D. *Let There Be Light.* Dinshah Health Society, 100 Dinshah Dr., Malaga, NJ 08328.

Dinshah, D. *The Spectro-Chrome System.* Dinshah Health Society, 100 Dinshah Dr., Malaga, NJ 08328

Hunt, R. *The Seven Keys to Color Healing: Diagnosis and Treatment Using Color.* New York: Harper and Row 1971.

Nelson, J. Guide to: *The Metaphysical Properties of Color.* 2572 46th St., San Diego, CA 92105.

For audio cassette color tapes related to the Dinshah method write: Jon Monroe 950 Agua Fria, Santa Fe, NM 87501 (505) 983-2823.

For color filters related to the Dinshah method contact: Multimedia Studio, 219 Shelby, Santa Fe, NM 87501.

Crystals

Alper, F. *Exploring Atlantis: Volumes 1 and 2.* Phoenix, AZ: Arizona Metaphysical Society, 1981.

Baer, R. and V. Bear. *Windows of Light: Quartz Crystals and Self-Transformaton.* San Francisco: Harper & Row, 1984.

Baer, R. and V. Baer. *The Crystal Connection: A Guidebook for Personal and Planetary Transformation.* San Francisco: Harper & Row, 1986.

Klinger-Raatz, U. *The Secrets of Precious Stones.* Lotus Light Publications, P.O. Box 2, Wilmot, WI 53192.

Lorusso, J. and J. Glick. *Healing Stoned: The Therapeutic Use of Gems and Minerals.* Albuquerque, NM: Brotherhood of Life, 1979.

Nelson, J. *Guide to: Crystals* 2572 46th St., San Diego, CA 92105.

Nelson, J. Guide to: *Metaphysical Properties of Stones* 2572 46th St., San Diego, CA 92105.

Raphaell, K. *Crystal Enlightenment: The Transforming Properties of Crystals and Healing Stones.* New York: Aurora Press, 1985.

Raphaell, K. *Crystal Healing: The Therapeutic Application of Crystals and Stones* Volume 2 New York: Aurora Press, 1987.

Chakra Balancing

Leadbeater, C.W. *The Chakras* 1927 (Reprint) Wheaton, Illinois: Theosophical Publishing House, 1977.

Motoyama, H. *Theories of the Chakras: Bridge to Higher Consciousness.* Wheaton, Illinois: Theosophical Publishing House, 1981.

Uhl, M. *Chakra Energy Massage.* Lotus Light Publications, P.O. Box 2, Wilmot, WI 53192.

Centering

Benson, H. *The Relaxation Response.* New York: Berkley Press, 1978.

Chia, Mantak. *Awaken Healing Energy Through The Tao* Santa Fe: Aurora Press, 1983.

Price, J. *Practical Spirituality.* Austin, Texas: Quartus Books, 1985.

CHAPTER 11

Airola, Paavo. *Are You Confused?.* Phoenix, AZ: Health Plus Publishing, 1974.

Airola, Paavo. *How to Get Well,* Phoenix, AZ: Health Plus Publishing, 1974.

Airola, Paavo. *How to Keep Slim Healthy and Young with Juice Fasting.* Phoenix, AZ: Health Plus Publishing, 1974.

Blackie, M. *The Patient, Not the Cure: The Challenge of Homeopathy.* Santa Barbara, CA: Woodbridge Press Publishing Co., 1978.

Cousens, G. *Spiritual Nutrition and the Rainbow Diet,* Boulder, CO: Cassandra Press, 1986.

Chang, S. *The Complete Book of Acupuncture.* Millbrae, CA: Celestial Arts, 1976.

Gerson, M. (1958) *A Cancer Therapy: The Cure of Advanced Cancer by Diet Therapy.* Bonita, CA: Gerson institute, 1986.

Kaptchuk, T. *The Webg That Has No Weaver. Understanding Chinese Medicine.* New York: Congdon & Weed, 1983.

Kulvinskas, Viktoras. *Survival Into the 21st Century.* Woodstock Valley, CT. Fairfield, Iowa: 21st Century Publications, 1975.

Laut, P. Rebirthing: *The Science of Enjoying All Your Life.* San Rafael, CA: Trinity Publishers.

Orr, L. and S. Ray. *Rebirthing in the New Age.* Berkely, CA: Celestial Arts, 1977.

Ray, S. *Celebration of Breath.* Berkeley, CA: Celestial Arts, 1983.

Wigmore, A. *A Hippocrates Diet.* Wayne, NJ: Avery Publishing Group, 1984.

CHAPTER 15

Baginski, B. and S. Sharamon. *Reiki – Universal Life Energy.* Mendocino, CA: Life Rhythm Publishing, 1988.

Gerson, M. (1958) *A Cancer Therapy – The Cure of Advanced Cancer by Diet Therapy.* Bonita, CA: Gerson Institute, 1986.

Hay, L. *You Can Heal Your Life* Farmingdale, NY: Coleman Publishing, 1984.

Kubler-Ross, E. *Death – The Final Stage of Growth.* Englewood Cliffs, NJ: Prentice Hall, 1975.

CHAPTER 16

Dychtwald, K. *Bodymind.* New York: Pantheon Books, 1977.

Lowen, A. *The Way to Vibrant Health – A Manual of Bioenergetic Exercises.* New York: Harper & Row, 1977.

Mindell, A. *Dreambody.* Santa Monica, CA: Sigo Press, 1982.

Rolf, I. *Rolfing: The Integration of Human Structures.* New York: Harper & Row, 1977.

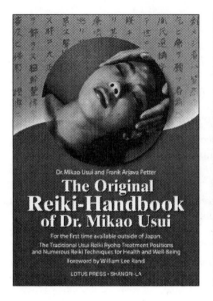

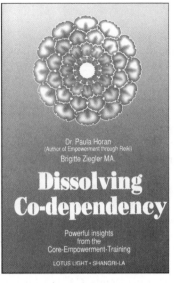

Dr. Mikao Usui and Frank A. Petter

The Original Reiki Handbook

The Traditional Usui Reiki Ryoho Treatment Positions and Numerous Reiki Techniques for Health and Well-Being

For the first time available outside of Japan: This book will show you the original hand positions from Dr. Usui's handbook. It has been illustrated with 100 colored photos to make it easier to understand. The hand positions for a great variety of health complaints have been listed in detail, making it a valuable reference work for anyone who practices Reiki. Now that the original handbook has been translated into English, Dr. Usui's hand positions and healing techniques can be studied directly for the first time. Whether you are an initiate or a master, if you practice Reiki you can expand your knowledge dramatically as you follow in the footsteps of a great healer.

80 pages, 100 photos, $ 14.95
ISBN 0-914955-57-8

Dr. Paula Horan · Brigitte Ziegler MA.

Dissolving Co-dependency

Powerful insights from the Core-Empowerment-Training

Dr. Paula Horan, a noted American psychologist, and her partner Brigitte Ziegler, a well know German seminar leader, are both Reiki masters, well versed in a wide variety of mind/body systems. They have put together a very powerful training to assist people in the dissolution of a lifetime of inappropriate thought, emotional, and behavioral patterns.The ulimate necessity of „waking up" in its truest sense, gives a very indepth background to the real workings of the human mind. Each chapter is followed by a simple exercise to help the reader assimilate each area of understanding. The book is for each individual who seeks a greater knowledge of self, with a sincere desire to get in touch with the core of being.

102 pages, $ 9,95
ISBN 0-941524-86-8

Herbs and other natural health products and information are often available at natural food stores or metaphysical bookstores. If you cannot find what you need locally, you can contact one of the following sources of supply.

Sources of Supply:

The following companies have an extensive selection of useful products and a long track-record of fulfillment. They have natural body care, aromatherapy, flower essences, crystals and tumbled stones, homeopathy, herbal products, vitamins and supplements, videos, books, audio tapes, candles, incense and bulk herbs, teas, massage tools and products and numerous alternative health items across a wide range of categories.

WHOLESALE:

Wholesale suppliers sell to stores and practitioners, not to individual consumers buying for their own personal use. Individual consumers should contact the RETAIL supplier listed below. Wholesale accounts should contact with business name, resale number or practitioner license in order to obtain a wholesale catalog and set up an account.

Lotus Light Enterprises, Inc.
PO Box 1008 ER
Silver Lake, WI 53170 USA
262 889 8501 (phone)
262 889 8591 (fax)
800 548 3824 (toll free order line)

RETAIL:

Retail suppliers provide products by mail order direct to consumers for their personal use. Stores or practitioners should contact the wholesale supplier listed above.

Internatural
PO Box 489 ER
Twin Lakes, WI 53181 USA
800 643 4221 (toll free order line)
262 889 8581 office phone
EMAIL: internatural@lotuspress.com
WEB SITE: www.internatural.com

Web site includes an extensive annotated catalog of more than 14,000 items that can be ordered "on line" for your convenience 24 hours a day, 7 days a week.

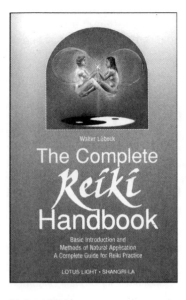

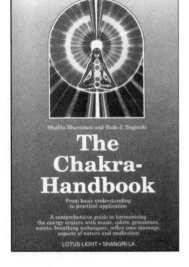

Walter Lübeck

The Complete Reiki Handbook

Basic Introduction and Methods of Natural Application. A Complete Guide for Reiki Practice

This handbook is a complete guide for Reiki practice and a wonderful tool for the necessary adjustment to the changes inherent in a new age. The author's style of natural simplicity, so beloved by the readers of his many bestselling books, wonderfully complements this basic method for accessing universal life energy. He shares with us, as only such a Reiki master can, the personal experience accumulated in his years of practice. The lovely illustrations of the different positons make the information as easily visually accessible, as does the author's direct and undogmatic style. This work also offers a synthesis of Reiki and many other popular forms of healing.

192 pages, $ 14.95
ISBN 0-941524-87-6

Shalila Sharamon and Bodo J. Baginski

The Chakra-Handbook

From basic understanding to practical application

Knowledge of the energy centers provides us with deep, comprehensive insight into the effects the subtle powers have on the human organism. This book vividly describes the functioning of the energy centers. For practical work with the chakras this book offers a wealth of possibilities: the application of sounds, colors, gemstones and fragrances with their own specific effects, augmented by meditation, breathing techniques, foot reflexology massage of the chakra points and the instilling of universal life energy. The description of nature experiences, yoga practices and the relationship of each indiviual chakra to the Zodiac additionally provides inspiring and valuable insight.

192 pages, $ 14,95
ISBN 0-941524-85-X